www.wadsworth.com

wadsworth.com is the World Wide Web site for Wadsworth and is your direct source to dozens of online resources.

At *wadsworth.com* you can find out about supplements, demonstration software, and student resources. You can also send e-mail to many of our authors and preview new publications and exciting new technologies.

wadsworth.com
Changing the way the world learns®

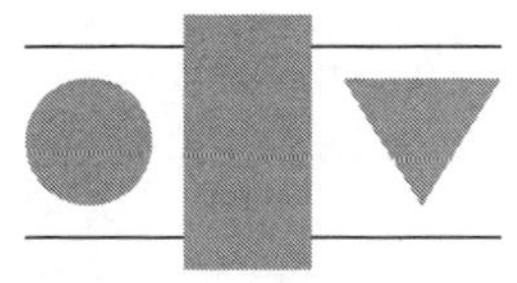

Basic Counseling Responses™ in Groups

A Multimedia Learning System for the Helping Professions

Hutch Haney
Seattle University

Jacqueline Leibsohn
Seattle University

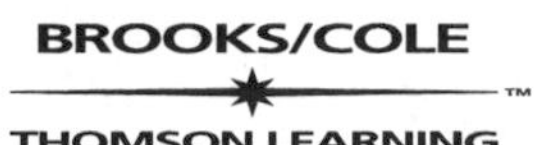

Australia • Canada • Mexico • Singapore • Spain
United Kingdom • United States

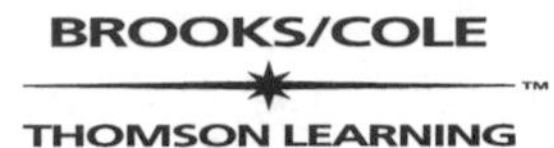

Counseling Executive Editor: Lisa Gebo
Assistant Editors: JoAnne von Zastrow, Susan Wilson
Editorial Assistant: Sheila Walsh
Marketing Manager: Caroline Concilla
Marketing Assistant: Jessica McFadden
Project Editor: Teri Hyde, Matthew Stevens
Print Buyer: Karen Hunt
Permissions Editor: Joohee Lee
Production Service: Penmarin Books
Photo Researcher: Connie Hathaway
Copy Editor: Cathy Baehler
Cover Designer: Margarite Reynolds
Compositor: Thompson Type
Indexer: Barbara Baxter
Cover Printer and Printer: Malloy Lithographing, Inc.

Printed in the United States of America

1 2 3 4 5 6 7 04 03 02 01 00

Library of Congress Cataloging-in-Publication Data

Haney, James Hutchinson.
Basic counseling responses in groups : a multimedia learning system for the helping professions / Hutch Haney, Jacqueline Leibsohn.
p. cm.
Includes bibliographical references and index.
ISBN 0-534-57573-0
1. Group counseling. 2. Group psychotherapy. 3. Group counseling—Problems, exercises, etc. 4. Group psychotherapy—Problems, exercises, etc. I. Leibsohn, Jacqueline. II. Title.
BF637.C6 H3195 2000
158'.35—dc21 00-034263

Wadsworth/Thomson Learning
10 Davis Drive
Belmont, CA 94002-3098
USA

For more information about our products, contact us:
Thomson Learning Academic Resource Center
1-800-423-0563
http://www.wadsworth.com

International Headquarters
Thomson Learning
International Division
290 Harbor Drive, 2nd Floor
Stamford, CT 06902-7477
USA

UK/Europe/Middle East/South Africa
Thomson Learning
Berkshire House
168-173 High Holborn
London WC1V 7AA
United Kingdom

Asia
Thomson Learning
60 Albert Street, #15-01
Albert Complex
Singapore 189969

Canada
Nelson Thomson Learning
1120 Birchmount Road
Toronto, Ontario M1K 5G4
Canada

This is dedicated to our families

MATT, ALEC, and JACOB LEIBSOHN

MARY ANNE and ADAM HANEY

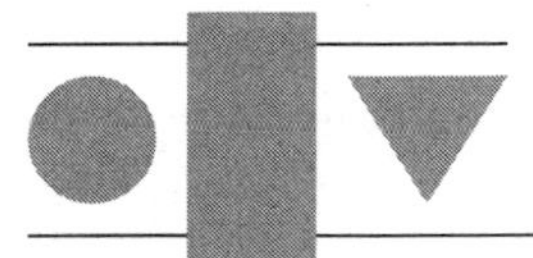

CONTENTS

Appendix A

Appendix B

Appendix C

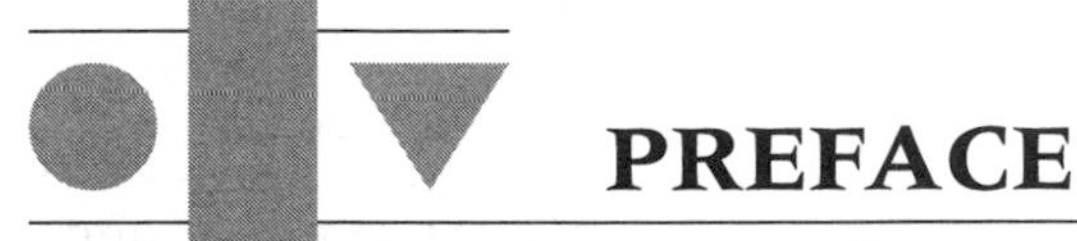

PREFACE

We believe in the power of groups. We have seen people make significant changes in their personal lives and in the ways that they interact with each other from participating in group counseling. The significant variable that makes the experience therapeutic is the trained group counselor. As counselor educators, we wanted a text that explained counseling responses in groups in a simplified, consistent language. We also wanted a text that emphasized intentionality and focus. Since it is our belief that observation is an excellent, nonthreatening learning opportunity, a videocassette, a CD-ROM, and a Web site are featured components of this package.

This package can stand alone. However, it is compatible with other group counseling texts, specifically, theory texts. This flexible package can be used as a complement to theory-based texts in a graduate program, as an introduction to group counseling at the undergraduate level, or for in-service training in a variety of situations. The fifteen responses in Part 2 are basic and generic and have been used in many counseling modalities.

Although we use the terms *counselor* and *group counseling,* this package is not limited to counseling; group work is done in all social services, schools, medical situations, and business. The principles and responses described herein can be applied to any group. We use the term *students* to refer to anyone using this package.

Many new and experienced counselors see groups as overwhelming. Conflict, for example, is almost always manifested in group counseling. This mirrors human conflict in almost any situation but can be intimidating to the group counselor. We felt that if students actually saw and experienced the role of the group counselor on the videocassette and the CD-ROM and could see how conflict, for example, is managed, they would embrace this power and the use of groups in their work.

Our biggest challenge in putting this package together was to avoid duplicating the many valuable texts that are more comprehensive and include chapters on all aspects of group work. We continually had to remind ourselves that our purpose was to demonstrate what the group counselor says in a group and how to identify that and to practice it. We did not want a text full of quotes from other authors, although we reference them when appropriate. We did quote Irvin Yalom's definitive *The Theory and Practice of Group Psychotherapy* (1995) relatively often because of its strong theoretical emphasis. We include sections on group development, ethics, diversity, and co-counseling because we felt that, even in brief, these issues needed to be part of a foundation for the descriptions and examples that follow. In Part 1, we included what we think are necessary sections on nonverbal responses, noncounseling responses, timing, group counselor responses, and responses to the difficult client.

We put an emphasis on client-generated responses, a phenomenon exclusive to groups. In the section on client responses in Part 1, we give examples from the videocassette and discuss our finding of the frequency of client-generated counseling responses in the groups that we taped. We also tracked the use of pronouns by clients to see if clients use "I" more frequently in the beginning of a group, then use "we" more often as they become more cohesive. The results are graphed in Appendix A and discussed in the text.

Basic Counseling Responses™ and *Basic Counseling Responses in Groups*™

In the worktext we previously authored, *Basic Counseling Responses* (Haney and Leibsohn, 1999), we presented a model for learning counseling responses that included fifteen counseling responses and associated intents and focuses. We have used those same fifteen responses with condensed definitions from *Basic Counseling Responses,* adding distinct examples and a discussion of how they are applicable to groups.

The focuses have also been expanded to include the focus on the total group and subgroups. We do not think that group counseling is individual counseling in a group setting; we believe that it is a distinct form of counseling, and the focus, while often on one or more individuals, must always return to the group. Believing that immediacy, or talking about the group process in the moment, is a significant variable in groups, we have given immediacy increased attention. We have also added the concept of focusing counseling responses in the context of the group itself.

We have also included two social work texts as references. *Social Work Practice with Groups* (1997) by Kenneth Reid is somewhat parallel in the social work profession to *Basic Counseling Responses* (1999). Reference to this is included in Table 1, Appendix A, Comparing *Basic Counseling Responses in Groups* to Responses/Skills of Other Models. Charles Zastrow's *Social Work with Groups* (1996) is a good source for group development and emphasizes variables of group work other than counseling. It is referenced in the group development section.

Note to Students and Instructors

If you have used *Basic Counseling Responses, Basic Counseling Responses in Groups* will be familiar. What makes *Basic Counseling Responses in Groups* unique is that each counseling response specifically explains the use of the respective responses in groups; the focus of counseling responses is considerably different and expanded; all of the exercises and references are group specific; and all video segments are of groups. In addition, the CD-ROM technology has advanced since the *Basic Counseling Responses* CD-ROM was made. Note also that we used the term *client* in focus identifications (for example, *client* feeling). In *Basic Counseling Responses in Groups* we use *individual* instead of *client* in the focus identifications to more clearly distinguish between one client in the group versus several clients in a group (individual feeling versus group feeling).

The Making of the *Basic Counseling Responses in Groups* Video

Our goal was to make a video of groups in action, but we did not want videos of counseling groups that were scripted and rehearsed. We believe group dynamics will happen when ordinary people interact without a script or rehearsal, with a counselor who makes clear, direct, simple counseling responses focused on the group.

We filmed eight sessions of both process groups and a curriculum-based structured group without rehearsals or scripts. Each group, even in the contrived environment of taping, exhibited group development from conflict and chaos to problem solving and cohesion. Attitudes and insight changed, and so did behavior.

The clients in these sessions are all volunteers. Adult clients are graduates or current students of a variety of programs within a university's college of education, including a counseling program. The adolescents are clients or students recruited from an agency and/or a school. The majority of clients did not know each other or their counselor before the sessions. Counselors are all graduates of a masters degree counselor education program. Some clients had previously participated in group counseling. Clients are identified by name, although many clients chose to use an alias. Clients and counselors represent a variety of ethnic and cultural backgrounds.

All groups were given a short orientation to the group experience. Adult clients chose the type of group that they wanted to be part of and wrote their personal goals for their group experience prior to the sessions. Most groups started with introductions and the sharing of goals, although these portions of the groups were edited out because of time constraints. Examples of goal statements can be found in Appendix A of the worktext. We did a follow-up study of clients, and we also used the unedited tapes to tally client responses and stage development as discussed in Appendix A. In addition, we report the results of a follow-up study of the clients in the five groups. All groups discussed confidentiality, and an example of one of these discussions is in transcript form in Appendix A. Clients knew that these discussions were "as if" the groups were confidential, which obviously, because they will be used for training, they are not.

Because of limited space, all sessions on the videocassette and the CD-ROM have been edited primarily for length. Editing was done with great care because we did not want to delete either the content or the process. Most edits were done when the content was redundant or not relevant to the primary theme of the group. For example, on the video with the adolescent boys, there was a great deal of discussion about sports and sports heroes. This was, of course, relevant to them and important for the counselor to allow. But for this demonstration video, we felt that those portions could be cut. Similar cuts were made in other sessions. The sequence of the sessions was not changed. Clients were not prompted, although counselors were on a few occasions, if a specific counseling response was needed for demonstration. We did not edit for language.

The videocassette starts with a segment explaining the *Basic Counseling Responses in Groups* (*BCRG*) model and how to use this learning system. It is followed by three complete sequential sessions of a women's group and a single session of an adolescent boys' group. The CD-ROM has clips from the women's group and clips from the boys' group, plus complete sessions of a graduate student group, a middle-school anger management group, and a co-counseled group of adults.

To the Student

Whether you are new to group counseling or an experienced group counselor, we believe that one is always a student of group counseling. This fascinating and complex counseling activity requires constant learning, experience, supervision, and consultation. We encourage you to look at groups you have participated in, whether it be your family or a classroom, and reflect on how groups have influenced your life. With this in mind, as you read the worktext, view the videocassette, and do the exercises, as well as using the CD-ROM and Web site, we think that you will see what we call the power of groups and how you as a student counselor can "counsel" this power to happen. If you have taken a counseling course for individual counseling, many of the things that you learned are applicable to group counseling. However, group counseling is distinct in that you are responding to a more complex client, which reflects far more diversity, intensity, and development than any single individual. We believe that this makes group counseling fascinating and of great therapeutic value.

Part 1 will give you an overall view of this model of learning counseling responses in groups and some of its variables, such as diversity, ethics, and group development. Part 2 defines and gives examples of fifteen counseling responses in groups. Part 3 contains exercises that give you the opportunity to identify and use the responses.

In addition to learning, identifying, and using responses, we hope that you will come to understand the therapeutic value of group counseling and what it is like to be a group counselor.

To the Instructor

The first segment of the videocassette is an introduction to the *Basic Counseling Responses in Groups* (BCRG) model and an explanation of the use of this learning system. This is a good starting place for both the instructor and the students.

The worktext, CD-ROM, and videocassette can precede, accompany, or follow the use of more theoretical texts on group counseling process and theory. We strongly recommend, especially in a graduate curriculum, that theory- and research-based texts be used as a foundation for learning specific counseling responses. Our experience as counselor educators is that many texts do an excellent job of describing group counseling, but few teach what the counselor can actually say in a group.

The exercises in the worktext and CD-ROM encourage beginning group counselors to both identify counseling responses, intents, and focuses used in the videos and to identify their own use of counseling responses. If you, as a counseling instructor, are familiar with our text *Basic Counseling Responses,* this is a similar teaching system.

In addition to describing specific counseling responses, their intents and focuses, we have included sections on group development, ethics, diversity, and co-counseling. These sections are not intended to replace the work of such authors as Yalom (1995) and Corey (2000) but are meant to reinforce the use of basic counseling responses in groups, the main focus of this work. We have included specialized bibliographies as references in Appendix B.

The worktext, videocassette, CD-ROM, and Web site can be used in a variety of ways in a variety of educational and training situations. The following are suggestions for their use:

1. The worktext includes information necessary for the completion of all exercises and should be read, discussed, and understood prior to starting the exercises. However, students can observe any session on the videocassette or CD-ROM before reading the text to get a sense of what group counseling sessions are like. This option may actually enhance their understanding of the information in the worktext.
2. The fifteen basic counseling responses in the worktext are in a suggested teaching order, but they can certainly be varied. The grouping of the counseling responses is also a way of teaching and learning the responses.
3. The videocassette has three complete sessions of a women's group, and a complete single session of an adolescent boys' group. There are exercises and transcripts in the worktext of these sessions. A description of the sessions is in Part 3. We think the value of this videocassette is that it can be shown to a large group of students and that it shows complete sessions.
4. The CD-ROM incorporates the exercises with clips from two sessions and three complete sessions. The worktext has transcripts of all sessions on the CD-ROM. The CD-ROM also has video examples of all 15 basic counseling responses, plus the intents and focuses. The CD-ROM is an excellent way for students to complete exercises on their own and to see a variety of counseling responses.

5. The Web site has a variety of resources and is updated regularly.
6. We recommend considering the following variables when deciding how to use the videocassette, CD-ROM, and Web site:
   a. Available technology
   b. Students' comfort level with technology
   c. Instructional situation

   We encourage instructors to try various combinations to determine what works best for both the students and instructor. The CD-ROM is designed primarily for individuals, whereas the videocassette can be used by individuals or small groups or in classroom demonstrations.
7. Exercises 1 and 2 for the videocassette are explained in Part 3 of the worktext. CD-ROM Exercises 1–5 are explained on the CD-ROM. A description of each group is also in Part 3. The exercises for the videocassette can be completed in the worktext using the Counseling Response Identification Format (CRIF) in both Appendix A and the CD-ROM file menu. The CD-ROM exercises are completed on the CD-ROM.
8. Advanced Exercises 1–5 are explained in the worktext only. They are offered for advanced student learning. These exercises can be done after completing the videocassette and CD-ROM exercises. They require a real or simulated group situation and supervision. The exercises allow students to apply the identification of response, intent, and focus to new sessions. Students can use the CRIF for identifying the responses, intents, and focuses for Advanced Exercises 1–5. Observers can watch the session, identify and record counseling responses used in the sessions and, in a debriefing session, tell the student/counselor what they observed. This increases the observation and identification skills of the observer, which are directly transferable to the role of counselor, and gives important feedback to the counselor.
9. We recommend that students start with Exercises 1 and 2 on the videocassette and then move to the CD-ROM. However, the number of completed exercises, the number of completed identifications in each exercise, and the order of the exercises should be based on such variables as the situation, student developmental levels, student progress, and instructor preferences. While all of the exercises build upon one another, they can be used in any order, either partially or completely, or in any way that meets the diverse teaching and learning situations of counselor education. If students choose to skip the videocassette exercises, they may want to watch these sessions before completing CD-ROM Exercises 1 and 2. CD-ROM Exercises 1 and 2 are clips from these complete sessions. Watching the complete sessions first on the videocassette may be helpful.
10. Reflection questions for videocassette Exercises 1 and 2 and the advanced exercises encourage students to discuss variables such as group development, ethics, diversity, client-generated counseling responses, and cocounseling. Instructors may want to add their own reflection questions.

The responses, intents, and focuses identified in the text and exercises by the authors are *only* suggestions. Students and instructors may have different interpretations of what the response, intent, or focus may be. Counseling is an art and not a science. What the counselor and group say and do is open for interpretation. We believe questioning and discussing what a counselor says is far more important than having a consensus about the definition or the label. We believe that these differences can lead to constructive discussions, including alternative identifications and alternative counselor responses. Throughout this worktext, emphasis is placed on *comparing* versus *judging*. Students are continually asked to identify responses, intents, and focuses to compare with the suggested identifications, with the understanding that there are no right and wrong identifications. We believe that this helps students understand that counseling is an art and that the way a counselor responds to a client is dependent on many variables and many interpretations.

If other models and theories of group counseling are used in a course or program, the terminology and concepts of these models and theories could be applied to the counseling sessions in this system. Table 1 in Appendix A compares the BCRG terminology to several other models.

Teaching a group counseling course involves more than having an appropriate text. It is recommended that this worktext, CD-ROM, videocassette, and Web site be used in concert with:

1. *Classroom lectures on various aspects of group counseling and the counseling profession.* The history of group counseling, counseling theories, and how they relate to groups, different kinds of groups, and different group populations, the current practice of group counseling, the distinctions between counseling and therapy, and ethics are topics all group counseling courses should include.
2. *Demonstration of counseling responses in groups.* Instructors should show how various responses are used within a group counseling session. Students should be encouraged to practice within the classroom for immediate feedback.
3. *Discussion of the use of counseling responses in groups with different clients in different settings.* Students should know the cultural and situational variables that influence the use of counseling responses. Specific gender, age, and cultural issues, for example, should be noted.
4. *Supplements:* Texts, journal articles, and related readings.

The format of a counseling course can be as follows:

1. Lecture and discussion on a specific group counseling topic.
2. Explanation and demonstration of selected counseling responses in groups.
3. Structured practice sessions in groups, preferably videotaped.
4. Feedback sessions with observers and instructors.
5. The review of practice sessions outside the classroom.
6. Periodic self-reflections and evaluations.

Using *Basic Counseling Responses* to Measure Student Learning

The *BCRG* videocassette/worktext exercises and the CD-ROM can be used to measure student learning. All exercises, but especially Videocassette Exercise 1 and CD-ROM Exercise 1, can be used as a pretest before the worktext is read or the videocassette or the CD-ROM is viewed. These exercises, or any other exercise, can also be used as a posttest after the worktext is read and the exercises are completed.

Another way of noting progress is by using the CD-ROM note boxes. Each CD-ROM exercise has a note box in which over a period of time the student can keep track of questions and ideas related to the exercises. These can be saved, printed, and forwarded via e-mail to other students and the instructor.

The reflection questions in the worktext that are associated with Videocassette Exercises 1 and 2 are another way in which the students can note their progress through this learning system.

Acknowledgments

We appreciate the inspiration and participation of students in the counseling programs at Seattle University. We are grateful to clients and counselors from community agencies and schools with which we are associated. We are especially grateful to Anna Fern for her help, to our colleagues at Seattle University, and to graduate students Paulette Pollard, Krista Coplin, Kara Ruotolo, and Toni Nicholes. Bill Good and Liz McKinney of Good Northwest and Jonathon and Billie Stratman of Reel Life Productions were our able partners in this project. Ever available and supportive was Lisa Gebo of The Wadsworth Group: Thanks again Lisa! Finally, we are indebted to the reviewers of this package.

Hutch Haney
Jacqueline Leibsohn

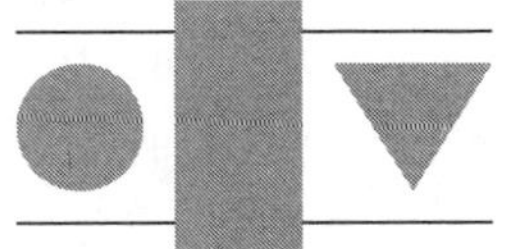

PART 1
Overview

This worktext, which accompanies a videocassette, CD-ROM, and Web site, leads the student through a process of learning group counseling responses, intents, and focuses. Part 1 is an overview of group counseling and includes issues such as group development, ethics, and diversity. In Part 2, fifteen group counseling responses are shown and identified, explained, and exemplified. In Part 3, exercises using the videocassette, CD-ROM, and Web site encourage the student and counselor to identify and demonstrate responses, intents, and focuses.

Philosophy and Language

Many group counseling texts use the terms *group leader* and *leadership* to describe the role of the counselor. In this text, *group counselor* will be consistently used to emphasize that the counselor *counsels* the group rather than *leads* the group. That is, the counselor responds to the group, even directs the group, but does not play the role as leader of the group. One goal of group counseling is to shift the responsibility of the group from the counselor to the group itself, further suggesting that a leadership definition of the counselor may not be descriptive.

Also, *response* will be used instead of *skill* because it more accurately describes the process of the counselor interacting with the group. The fifteen basic counseling responses described in Part 2 are considered generic responses because they have been used in a variety of counseling modalities. Their use does not preclude the use of other counseling interventions and techniques. Any response from a counselor should be consistent with the philosophy of the counselor—grounded in theory and research, relevant to the content, issues, and development of the group, and appropriate to the dynamics of the group membership.

The term *counselor* may include other professionals, such as teacher, nurse, pastoral counselor, social worker, or any other person who is in the role of *counseling* a group. Especially in references, *counselor* will be used interchangeably with *therapist,* as will *counseling* and *therapy*. Individuals in a group will be referred to in this text as clients or members. However, there are many exceptions. For example, in a school, the clients may be called students, and in an agency, the clients may be called consumers. Yalom (1995), quoted often in this worktext, calls them patients.

Not all groups are specifically called *counseling* groups. For example, an anger management group in a school may be considered a curriculum-based group. Counseling responses can be incorporated into the curriculum of this group to help the students become more aware of their process and interactions. Group 4/students on the videocassette is an example of an anger management group. Groups may be task oriented, designed for specific populations, have open or closed membership, focus on a specific theme or have a problem to solve. Groups vary in the length of each session, the frequency of sessions, and the number of participants. The term *group* in this text will refer to an average size group of seven or eight clients, though the responses and many of the concepts presented can apply to couples or triads. Even a group of two clients presents a different dynamic than a single client. The variables and combinations of variables are endless.

A significant component of group counseling is that the focus is on the clients, not a topic or issue. Therefore, one common denominator is that the group counselor always brings the focus back to what is happening in the group or how the group is responding to what has been presented. The *focus* indicates to whom the response is directed; whether at the experience, thought, behavior or feeling; as well as the immediacy and context of the response. The *intent* is what the counselor wants to accomplish by acknowledging, exploring, or challenging the group when making a response.

Basic Counseling Responses in Groups

The counseling responses that a group counselor makes to a group may resemble counseling responses made to an individual. The type of response (QUESTIONING or EMPATHIZING, for example) will be the same, though the language, intent, and focus for a group may be different.

Intents of *Basic Counseling Responses in Groups*

It is important, though often difficult, to be intentional when making counseling responses. Counselors learn to respond from observation and practice, but the "why" of those responses is often elusive, even in retrospect. The purpose of naming the intent of a counseling response is to encourage the counselor to be more aware of his or her role. This increases the likelihood that the counselor is responding both appropriately and therapeutically. The group counselor can respond directly to the group, a subgroup or an individual with the following three intents:

- To acknowledge what has been said or heard in the group both verbally and nonverbally is a primary intent of many counseling responses. Acknowledging shows interest and respect, and models communication factors that facilitate interpersonal communication. ATTENDING is a counseling response that acknowledges.
- To explore what has been said in the group by using, the counseling response of CLARIFYING, for example, is done to help clients gain new information or insight by being more concrete and precise.
- To challenge a group is to give a different perspective or to ask the group for a different perspective. The intent to challenge is often seen as confrontational because it encourages the group, or individuals in the group, to reassess their situation or consider a change of behavior

or belief. REFRAMING, DIRECTING, or NOTING A DISCREPANCY are examples of counseling responses that challenge.

The counselor, using the responses of DIRECTING or QUESTIONING, can challenge the whole group, part of the group, or an individual to say or do something directly to the group, part of the group, or an individual. This is done in lieu of the counselor making the response and can only be done in a group. The intent is to challenge some group members to challenge other members of the group.

"I would like for members of the group who do not agree to tell the other members how they are feeling?'

DIRECTING to challenge subgroup behavior

"What do the three of you observe happening between these two?"

QUESTIONING to challenge subgroup behavior

To challenge any part of the group to challenge any other part of the group, the counselor must give up some control; the counselor cannot control what members of the group will say to each other, especially when being asked to challenge. This trust within the group can be based on the belief that a noncounselor response may be more important than a counselor-generated response (see Client Responses, page17).

The counselor's intent may be perceived as different from the intent of both the clients in a group and anyone observing the group. The counselor may intend to acknowledge the group behavior by saying, "I notice that many members of the group are nodding their heads"; but certain members of the group may feel that the counselor is challenging their behavior in the group. In this case, the counselor may have more than one intent. By acknowledging a certain behavior, the counselor may also want the client to explore that particular behavior. When identifying the intent of a response, the primary intent should be named.

These descriptions of the intents are specific to identifying counseling responses. However, the intent of every counseling response should be to promote factors that are therapeutic, and meet the goals of the group, whether they be set by the group itself or those offering the group. For example, the counselor may say, "How does the group feel about the anger that was just expressed?" using the counseling response of QUESTIONING to challenge the group. While at the same time, the response is inclusive of two of Yalom's (1995) therapeutic factors, "development of socializing techniques" and "interpersonal learning"; and helps meet the goal of the group, which may be to learn to manage anger.

Five things should be remembered about intents:

1. The intent of a counseling response may not always be clear to observers.
2. It may be more important to process what the intent was, than have a precise answer. (Intents are easier to see in retrospect.)
3. It is important for the counselor to know how their responses are received by their clients through attending or questioning; clients may perceive the intent differently than what was meant by the counselor.
4. The intent to challenge members to challenge the group is powerful and should be used with discretion.
5. Identifying the counselor's intent is speculative; only the counselor can be sure of the intent. However, being speculative increases awareness of the intent and can help students identify their own intents.

Focuses of *Basic Counseling Responses in Groups*

In the *Basic Counseling Responses in Groups* (*BCRG*) model, determining the focus of a counseling response in groups involves identifying:

- *Who*: group, subgroup or individual;
- *What*: experience, thought, feeling or behavior;

plus the additives of

- *Where*: context
- *When*: immediacy

The focus of the counseling response is one primary characteristic that can distinguish individual counseling from group counseling. In individual counseling, the focus should generally be on the client. In group counseling, the focus can be on an individual, a part of the group, or the group as a whole (the *who*). As in individual counseling, the counselor can also focus on experience, thought, behavior, or feeling (the *what*). Additionally, the counselor can sharpen the focus of the counseling response by stating the context of the group (the *where*), a dynamic that does not exist in individual counseling. The counselor can also emphasize the immediacy of the interaction, the "here and now" (the *when*), as a counselor would with an individual.

Who

The group counselor has the option to direct the counseling response to an individual, part of the group (subgroup), or to the group as a whole. The focus on the entire group, using the terms *the group* or *you* is explained by Yalom (1995).

> Some leaders choose to focus primarily or entirely on mass group phenomena. These leaders refer, in their statement, to the "group" or "we" or "all of us." They attempt to clarify the relationship between the "group" and its primary task, that is, the investigation of intermember—and I include the leader here—relationships, or between the "group" and one of its members, a subgroup, the leader, or some shared concern (p. 177).

A note about the use of *we* by the counselor: While focusing on the entire group is a significant variable unique to group counseling, the counselor is generally considered *with* the group, but not *in* the group. Therefore, it is recommended that the counselor not use *we* or *all of us* if the counselor does not want to imply inclusiveness. There are, no doubt, many exceptions and counselor preferences that may contradict this recommendation.

What

The counselor also determines on what the focus will be placed. The focus can be on the experience of the group—what is going on in the group right now—or more specifically on the thoughts, feeling, or behavior of the group or subgroup. "What does the group think about . . . ?" "I notice that some members of the group are feeling tired" and "Several people are smiling" are respective examples of focus. Experience is the broader focus; the sharpest focus in a group is on thoughts, feelings, or behaviors.

TABLE 1: FOCUSES: WHO AND WHAT

WHO/WHAT	EXPERIENCE	THOUGHT	FEELING	BEHAVIOR
INDIVIDUAL	"You are experiencing some difficulty in the group."	"What do you think is going on?"	"You feel that there is a connection between your feeling and the group situation?"	"You laugh when you say that."
SUBGROUP	"How are the other members of the group experiencing this?"	"What do the two of you think about what they said?"	"Some members of the group are feeling sad."	"Several people are smiling."
GROUP	"How does the group experience this silence?"	"What does the group think about this?	"How does the group feel about the silence?"	"I notice that the group is very quiet."

Table 1 shows twelve options available to the counselor for identifying the *who* and the *what* of the focus.

Where

By focusing on the context of the group, the counselor uses the power of the group situation that is not available in a nongroup situation. Even with the focus on an individual client, it is often within the context of the group: "How is it for you to share that *with the group*?" In focusing on an individual, the counselor can differentiate between making a counseling response that is individually focused verses making a counseling response that is individually focused in the context of the group. For example:

> "Sally, how is it to talk about this feeling?"
> QUESTIONING to explore individual feeling

versus

> "Sally, how is it to talk about this feeling in the group?"
> QUESTIONING to explore individual feeling in *context*

The same is true in responding to the group or a subgroup, by adding "in the group." For example:

> "How is it for the three of you to feel stuck?"
> QUESTIONING to explore subgroup feeling

versus

> "How is it for the three of you be stuck in this group?"
> QUESTIONING to explore group feeling in *context*

When

The counselor also chooses the time frame to focus on the past, future, or present. Most counseling responses are in the present tense: "The group is . . . ." The group seems . . . ." Does the group . . . ?" Immediacy is more than just the present tense. It has to do with the present moment or the immediate events of the session, and clearly defining the present moment.

Therefore, in addition to choosing the *who* and the *what,* and possibly adding the *where,* the counselor can add the focus of immediacy, the *when.* The focus can be on the group feeling with or without immediacy. For example:

> "The group seems to be experiencing some sadness."

versus

> "The group seems to be experiencing some sadness *right now.*"

These examples show the difference between an implied immediacy and a clearly stated immediacy. When the counselor says, "The group is feeling," the implication is that the counselor is talking about the immediate moment. But by saying "right now" the counselor takes the response one step further; the counselor makes the group more aware that this is something happening now, not several minutes ago or in a previous session.

Additives of Context and Immediacy

The two additives of context and immediacy are words the counselor uses to further sharpen the focus of the counseling responses. The counselor can emphasize the context of the group by saying, for example, "in this group," and the counselor can denote the current time frame by adding "right now." These additives take advantage of the group environment (context) and the here and now aspect of the group experience (immediacy).

Both of the additives must be *stated, not implied.* By explicitly stating the context or immediacy of the group experience, the counselor makes it clear to the group that what they are saying, doing, and feeling is grounded in this place and time. Even though this may be implied, it may not be obvious. By adding these focus variables, the counselor makes the place and time more obvious, thus making the focus of the counseling response clearer and sharper. For example, the context additive is clear if the counselor says, with the focus on the group, "How is the group reacting to what is happening *in the group*?" However, If the counselor says, "How is the group reacting to what is happening?" the identification of the context additive is not as overt, though the implication is that the counselor is referring to the group itself. In both using and identifying context and immediacy, all examples of both throughout *Basic Counseling Responses in Groups* will be in responses that *state rather than imply* the context and/or immediacy.

The therapeutic value of focusing on immediacy in a group is best described by Yalom (1995):

> This focus greatly facilitates the development and emergence of each member's social microcosm. It facilitates feedback, catharsis, meaningful self-disclosure, and the acquisition of socializing techniques (p. 129) . . . the effective use of the here-and-now requires two steps: the group lives in the here-and-now, and it also doubles back on itself; it performs a self-reflective loop and examines the here and now behavior that has just occurred (p. 130).

TABLE 2: WHEN: THE FOCUS ADDITIVE OF IMMEDIACY

TENSE			IMMEDIACY
PAST	FUTURE	PRESENT	"AT THIS MOMENT"
"The group felt scared." EMPATHIZING to acknowledge group feeling	"The group will feel scared." EMPATHIZING to acknowledge group feeling	"The group feels scared." EMPATHIZING to acknowledge group feeling	"The group feels scared right now." EMPATHIZING to acknowledge group feeling with immediacy

Thus, the counselor not only emphasizes what is happening in the group in the immediate moment, but also encourages the group to reflect on how the group is experiencing the moment. This is the self-reflective loop dynamic noted by Yalom.

The additives of immediacy and context can be used together. For example:

"You are feeling awkward sharing this in this group right now."
EMPATHIZING to acknowledge individual feeling with immediacy in context

The counselor can focus on more than one *who* and more than one *what.* For example:

"I notice that Bill and several other members of the group are moving around in their seats."
GIVING FEEDBACK to acknowledge individual and subgroup behavior

"There seems to be a discrepancy between how the group is feeling and how the group is acting."
NOTING A DISCREPANCY to challenge group feeling and behavior

Definition of Group Counseling

Group counseling can be defined as *clients interacting with each other to increase their awareness of themselves as individuals and participants in a group; to explore possibilities to change; and take action regarding the changes within the group. Using counseling responses, the counselor increases awareness by acknowledging what is happening in the group, facilitates possibilities of change by exploring those possibilities, and generating action by challenging the group.*

Group counseling is counseling with a consistent immediacy focus, emphasizing the interaction between individuals as it happens within the context of the group. As a trained professional, the counselor keeps the focus on the group as much as possible with the belief that the dynamics of group behavior and development are the most important therapeutic factor in a group.

Group counseling is NOT individual counseling in a group setting. Group counseling is NOT teaching an identified body of knowledge. Group counseling is NOT a support group for individuals with like situations led by a person that is not a trained counselor. However, in most group counseling situations, it is likely that some focus will be on individuals, some sharing of information will take place, and a sense of support will develop.

The goals of each counseling group are going to be as varied as the goals of each individual client. Group goals will vary within the group, and may not coincide with the goals of the counselor.

Goals should be discussed in prescreening and during the group sessions. The goal of a counseling group is not necessarily the end stage of a developmental model or the attainment of the group's goals. While group cohesion, for example, may be a valued goal, not all groups become cohesive. However, the process of moving toward it—the movement—may be as important as getting there.

The Group Counselor

The group counselor must believe that groups are therapeutic. For example, the counselor can believe that how clients respond in the group is similar to how clients respond in other group settings, and what clients learn in the group is transferable to situations outside of the group. Yalom (1995) calls this the client's social microcosm:

> Given enough time, the group members will begin to be themselves: they will interact with the group members as they interact with others in their social sphere, will create in the group the same interpersonal universe they have always inhabited (p. 28) . . . behavior learned in group is eventually carried over into the patient's social environment (p. 43).

The group counselor has more responsibility in planning and implementing a group because more people are involved and more logistics are considered. The group counselor must do tasks not required of the counselor of individuals such as prescreening, setting norms, and conducting appropriate group activities.

The group counselor must also have the personal attributes and professional abilities necessary to all counselors. Gladding (1999), in discussing the counselor, gives a definition of group counseling:

> . . . Group leaders should recognize that a number of group skills are the same as those displayed in working with individuals. For example, group leaders must be empathetic, caring and reflective. At the same time, a number of special skills are unique to group leaders, and leaders must always keep in mind that a group is more than just a collection of individuals. It is an interactive system in which attention to one group member or topic will have an impact on all group members and the group process (p. 83).

The group counselor must be comfortable with the conflictual and paradoxical nature of group counseling. The following quote explains what is meant by conflict and paradox. [Kottler (1994), citing Benne (1968) and Berg and Smith (1990).]

1. Groups are among the safest and the most dangerous environments.
2. Does the group exist for individuals (autonomy) or do the members exist for the group (cohesion)?
3. Diversity among members allows for breadth of input and yet makes things more prone to conflict.
4. If the group leader supports both members in conflict, the fighting escalates.
5. Mutual dependency is necessary before independence can develop.
6. Boundaries within the group both encourage and limit actions by members.
7. Members are encouraged to become worse before they get better.

The group counselor must also be willing to be present to the entire group. Note that Yalom's (1995) explanation of *presence* also adds that it is the quality that clients remember:

> . . . You do by being, by being there with the patient. Presence is the hidden agent of help in all forms of therapy. Patients, looking back on their therapy rarely remember a single interpretation you made, but they always remember your presence, that you were there with them (p. 96).

Group counseling is a paradox. On one hand, it is very different than individual counseling because the focus is on more people and the dynamics of the group are often more influential than the counselor. On the other hand, the group counselor can respond to the group the same way an individual counselor may respond to an individual. For example, if the group counselor does not know what counseling response to use in a group, one might consider what could be said to an individual client. For example, when there is no verbal interaction in the group, the counselor feels a need to do something. With an individual, the counselor may ask a question, or comment on the silence. The same can be done in the group: "How would the group like to deal with the silences?" (QUESTIONING to challenge group behavior.)

There is a tendency for the group counselor to respond as a teacher. The very number of members in a group suggests the counselor assumes the role that a teacher may assume in a classroom. The counselor may prepare a valuable educational component, such as information about anger management or structured exercises and may rely on classroom techniques and procedures. However, these are not considered counseling responses and don't distinguish the counseling experience from an educational experience. For example, a group of adolescents are in a "children of divorce group." The group is co-counseled by a classroom teacher and a school counselor. In the first meeting the students raise their hands before they talk, as they have dutifully learned. The teacher says, "You don't have to raise your hands in the group"; the counselor says, "I notice that the members of this group raise their hands before they talk." (GIVING FEEDBACK to acknowledge group behavior.) The teacher is doing what teachers do, and most often should do: telling the group what they can or should do. The counselor on the other hand, gives feedback to the group with the expectation that the group may decide a norm for themselves regarding their interaction. Both responses are right for the respective roles, but are based on a different perception of the counseling versus educational nature of the group and the goals and objectives relative to those roles. Both the counselor and teacher may find this teacher/counselor differential helpful when deciding the nature of their responses.

Group Development

The central focus of many group counseling texts is group development. Group development is a significant variable in the group and mirrors how people relate and change both inside and outside the therapeutic group setting. Stage theories abound; any and all are useful. Several models will be referenced as they apply to the groups used for this learning package.

In *The Different Drum, Community Making and Peace*, Peck (1987), says, "So it is that groups assembled deliberately to form themselves into communities routinely go through certain stages" (p. 86). The stages described by Peck are not only very parallel to other models, but the terms, especially *pseudocommunity* and *chaos* and *emptiness* can be very descriptive of the early development of a group. Peck speaks of emptiness as "the bridge" between chaos and community:

> As they enter the stage of emptiness the members of the group come to realize—sometimes suddenly and sometimes gradually—that their desire to heal, convert, or otherwise 'solve' their interpersonal differences is a self-centered desire for comfort through the obliteration of these differences (p. 98).

Thus, emptiness may look like conflict and clients struggle with themselves and each other to let go of their need to control and move toward cohesiveness as a group. The beginning of Group 2/boys is an example of chaos. Yet, within this chaos there are indications that the group is aware of its "groupness" and may be starting to enter this sense of emptying. Thomas (2.42) says, "Sorta weird, cause nobody got nothin', everybody say, nobody wants to talk about it. Nobody can agree on anything." Also, early in the development of this group, in the discussion about what to talk about, there is the acknowledgement that to talk about something personal is scary: Counselor (2.75): "What would happen in the group if we talked about something personal?"; Rick (2.76) "Probably be scary." This fear of intimacy is what Peck (1987) suggests that clients must empty themselves of to, ironically, obtain intimacy in the group.

The final session of Group 1/women has many examples acknowledging the community and cohesiveness of this group. One example is what Jean (1c.12) says, "And, and then because of that I think it was hard work that we did that and then when we really had to do some of the hard stuff in the group, for me that trust that I had experienced and that I think we all felt it was . . . " Another example is in Group 4/students, the anger management group. Andre says, "Um, I like just knowing that I'm not the only one that has these problems, like there are four other people here, five other people that have these problems. The same problems as I do." Kyle also expressed a sense of universality, as noted by Yalom (1995): "In the therapy group, especially in the early stages, the disconfirmation of a patient's feeling of uniqueness is a powerful source of relief" (p. 6).

Groups, while following general patterns of behavior shown in the models listed in Table 3 rarely move clearly from step to step. Yalom (1995) states, "The boundaries between phases are not clearly demarcated, nor does the group permanently graduate from one phase" (p. 303). This is echoed by Corey (1995), "There is considerable overlap between stages, and once a group moves to an advanced stage of development, there may be temporary regressions to earlier developmental stages" (p. 130). With equal wisdom, a third-grade student noted that her loss and grief group "worked in waves." This comment was in response to the group counselor noting a shift in the group energy.

As a group develops, it is likely to become more group-centered, more autonomous, and less dependent on the counselor. This is noted by Yalom (1995): "If the group continues to regard the therapist as the sole source of aid, the group fails to achieve an optimum level of autonomy and self-respect" (p. 125). An example of group dependency on the counselor appears early in the adolescent boys group, Group 2/boys (2.7), when Thomas says to the counselor, "Yeah, you're supposed to run this thing." An example of the group becoming more independent and less dependent on the counselors, is when Amy, from Group 3/graduates, says (3.24), "I have to be honest and say that it's good for me to hear a different perspective, but although I have to admit, the fact that you guys (the counselors) are feeling frustrated means less to me than if these guys (the group) were frustrated." Challenging the group leader is often a characteristic of the transition stage (Corey, 2000): "If members are to become free of their dependency on the leader that is characteristic of the initial group stage, the leader must allow and deal directly with these revealing challenges to his or her authority" (p. 108). When Barbara and Sue (1b.21–1b.33) question the counselor's "pushing" of Barbara regarding her anger, these clients are challenging the counselor.

Sometimes a significant change in the group or in an individual's behavior in the group can be seen. In Group 2/boys, Thomas becomes aware of what it means to interrupt others by understanding what it means to be interrupted himself (2.345–2.352): The counselor (2.510) says to Thomas, "How do you feel about being cut off?" and Thomas says (2.511)" . . . It makes you feel sort of bad because . . . ." Later, Thomas says (2.577), ". . . It's sort of good when they (Rick and

Wallace) told me what they were feeling 'cause if they didn't say what they felt like, I would continue to interrupt them and they could end up getting really mad."

In the latter stage of a group, members with some perspective are able to express what they have learned from the experience. Rachel, Group 4/students, expressed this type of reflection, "I think for me the group has helped me realize like what I am doing sometimes when I get really mad at people, I don't even realize it at first, what I am doing."

Also later in group development, members are able to articulate the experience of termination as Vee does at (1c.17), Group1/women, "I was just thinking there is a sense of sadness when we're trying to talk about where we were and how it has been, but as I kept hearing everyone talk it seems like the good-byes are not going to be final."

In *Social Work with Groups*, Zastrow (1997) compares the stages of groups with the stages of working with individuals (p. 17):

Groups	*Individuals*
Intake	Intake
Selection of members	
Assessment and planning	Assessment and planning
Group development and intervention	Intervention
Evaluation and termination	Evaluation and termination

Zastrow's model emphasizes issues such as selection of group members, as part of the stages of group development. In a discussion on this, Zastrow cites the Garland, Jones, and Kolodny model of preaffiliation, power and control, intimacy, differentiation, and separation. Zastrow says,

> The differentiation stage is analogous to a healthy functioning family in which the children have reached adulthood and are now becoming successful in pursuing their own lives. Relationships are more between equals, and members are mutually supportive and able to relate to each other in more rational and objective ways (p. 21).

Zastrow also cites the Tuckman model, which is familiar to most group counselors: forming, storming, norming, performing, and adjourning. He also notes the nonsequential, nondevelopmental Bales model:

> Bales asserted that groups continue to seek an equilibrium between task-oriented work and emotional expressions, in order to build better relationship among members. . . . Bales asserts that groups tend to oscillate between these two concerns (p. 22).

With the belief that group development, while not necessarily a step-by-step process, is important to know, and believing that group development is observable, counselors are encouraged to understand how their particular group moves through a developmental process for three reasons:

1. Knowing where the group is can help the counselor give appropriate feedback: "I notice that the group members are feeling some tension with each other."
2. By comparing the group to a developmental model, the counselor can question whether the movement of the group needs to be addressed. For example, if the group is not moving toward any sense of cohesion the counselor may feel that the group needs some direction: "I wonder if the group could talk about how they feel about each other?"
3. Counselors need to know about group development to understand that many of the phenomena, for example, conflict between members and challenging the counselor being two of

them, are natural occurrences of most groups. Yalom (1995) notes: "a knowledge of broad developmental sequence will provide you with a sense of mastery and direction in a group and prevent you from feeling confused and anxious . . ." (p. 294).

Tracking the Development of the *BCRG* Groups

There are many examples in the five groups on the videocassette and CD-ROM concerning the stage development of the various models in Table 3. Group 2/boys and the ending of Group 3/graduates are examples of conflict. The final stage of Group 1/women, Group 2/boys, and Group 4/students expresses the value of the group experience. Group 5/adults shows how several of the stages happen within one group session. To determine the development of the five groups, the pronouns group members used were tracked and graphed in the unedited versions of the eight sessions (see Appendix A, Charts 1–5). This was done with the hypothesis that clients would change their use of pronouns as the groups developed. Clients might be expected to use "I" during the initial stages of the group when members are not feeling part of the group. As conflict arises, "you" statements will become more frequent because members are interacting more with each other. "We" statements will occur more as the group moves toward cohesion and starts to work as a group. Yalom (1995), regarding cohesiveness and the "we" says,

> Several hundred research articles exploring cohesiveness have been written, many with widely varying definitions. In general, however, there is agreement that groups differ from one another in the amount of "groupness" present. Those with a greater sense of solidarity, or "we-ness," value the group more highly and will defend it against internal and external threat. Such groups have a higher rate of attendance, participation and mutual support, and will defend the group standards much more than groups with less esprit de corps (p. 48).

It was anticipated that the use of "I" would be significantly more prevalent throughout the sessions because most clients start any sentence about themselves with "I." The use of "I" included using "you" or "we" when the clients were clearly talking about themselves. "You" statements also included any reference to another person in the group. "We" statements included statements using terms such as *the group* or *us*.

Chart 1 of Group 1/women in Appendix A exemplifies the anticipated result of this data collection. In the middle of the second of three groups, the "you"s increased and the "I"s decreased. This reflects the tension the group experienced as it worked through the group's responses to Barbara's anger. Expressions of the "we-ness" of the group occurred at the end of the final session. The rise in "I" at the end reflects the individual statements of each member regarding their experience of the group. It might be surmised that this group followed a more anticipated pattern of group development, or group movement, because it met three different times. Group 3/graduates followed a similar pattern, but the one and only session ended when the group was experiencing some conflict with the counselors and some tension with each other. Note the sharp decrease of "I"s and increase of "you"s that reflects this shift. Group 5/adults also showed a pattern of decreasing "I"s, rising "we"s and "you"s that peak in the middle. Again, though this group met only once, the CD-ROM session and the transcripts seem to confirm this pattern. Group 2/boys and Group 4/students do not follow the pattern. Though they reflect the same higher frequency of "I"s and lower frequency of "we"s, no clear patterns emerge. Perhaps adults have a more predictable pattern of group development, while adolescents express various

TABLE 3: STAGE MODELS FOR GROUP DEVELOPMENT

	MODEL					
	Peck	Corey	Yalom	Garland, Jones, Kolodny	Tuckman	*BCRG*
STAGE	Pseudo community	Initial: Orientation and Exploration	Initial	Pre-affiliation	Forming	"I"
	Chaos	Transition: Dealing with Resistance	Conflict	Power and control	Storming Norming	"You"
	Emptiness					
	Community	Working: Cohesion and Productivity	Cohesive	Intimacy	Performing	"We"
		Final: Consolidation and termination	Advanced	Differentiation Separation	Adjourning	

stages of group development inconsistently. This was true of their use of counseling responses as well. However, both Group 2/boys and Group 4/students expressed, just not predictably, conflict within "you" statements and cohesion in "we" statements.

Table 3 parallels several stage models with the *BCRG* model "I," "you," and "we" concepts.

Diversity

Groups by their very nature are diverse. More than one person means more than one set of values, experiences, and expressions. Groups are formed by and for many populations: older adults or individuals with chemical dependencies are two examples. But, no matter how alike clients in a group may appear, clients are from different families and parts of the country, and larger cultures and different parts of the world. An apparent homogeneous group may have as many differences within the group regarding disclosure, interaction, and affective expression as a group that is a combination of other cultures, genders, and families. Conversely, no matter how differently clients in a group may appear, they are likely to share certain values, feelings, and experiences.
Consider the following:

- Members of the group can share their apparent differences with the group; encourage all clients to do so. Sexual orientation, gender, and belief systems are only some of the variables

that may need to be acknowledged in addition to, or as part of, a culture. Encourage the expression of difference with the understanding that universal values and experiences might be discovered. The values regarding behavior, feeling, and thoughts are manifest in a group because their differences are contrasted as group members self-disclose. As similarities are also acknowledged, the concept of universality as a therapeutic factor (Yalom, 1995) is reinforced.
- The group counselor must be open to learning about diverse variables, but the counselor does not have to be the expert; the counselor's expertise cannot compete with the expertise of the clients who have lived with diverse variables. Individuals are the experts in the variables that influence their lives; use them as a resource. Referring to her own ethnicity, Maria (4.49) says, "I wouldn't care if people ask me. They always assume. Nobody ever asks me." Referring to her own cultural experience relative to the expression of anger, Linda (1b.68) first says, "But I live in a world where things are not fair and you experience it a lot and you don't get angry every time, but because the experience is so frequent you tend to exhibit anger more than other people would"; and then, at (1b.74), "I have a competency here . . . "
- Counseling responses are relatively atheoretical and generic, but counselors must be aware of how their responses are perceived by clients and explore this in the group. The values that clients hold may be a significant variable of diversity. Self-disclosure, for example, may not be a value that all clients share and, therefore, may have an influence on the group dynamics.

One more suggestion, though simplistic, is often forgotten: Never assume. Groups vary as much within themselves as with each other. Words that are used to define larger groups of people may be defined differently by members of the same identified group. Smaller groups, like families, are cultures within themselves and share and promote their own values. Differences and similarities are often not visible; people have feelings and values that are not evident or expressed and those feelings and values can never be assumed.

Ethics

Group counselors must be aware of: (a) the codes of ethics, such as *Ethical Guidelines for Group Counselors* published by the Association for Specialists in Group Work (ASGW), that apply to group counseling and (b) the legal consideration of group work. Three issues are especially important in group counseling: setting norms, confidentiality, and safety. While it may be valuable for groups to set some of their own norms regarding other group aspects, confidentiality and safety should be set by the counselor and be regarded as nonnegotiable. Both confidentiality and safety, and other norms specific to the group, should be discussed in prescreening or preeducation.

Safety is often an issue because of the volatile nature of some groups, especially while in conflict. Depending on the nature of the group, the counselor may be required, either prior to the group or during a session, to set specific norms for group behavior ranging from no advice giving to no hitting. Clients may need to be educated on how to give feedback or how to interact during conflict. The consequences of violating norms, whether determined by the counselor or the group, must be clear and enforced.

Morganett (1990), notes "one of the leader's important roles is to help establish positive norms for expression and conduct in a group" (p. 8). She differentiates between explicit norms, or ground rules, that are developed by the counselor and added to by the members. They may be written and unwritten rules, such as arriving on time and being respectful. She also cautions, "be aware of emerging norms in your group so that you can support positive norms and eliminate negative ones" (p. 8).

The group counselor has less control about what happens in and out of the group counseling session than in individual counseling. Group counselors can do everything possible to inform and insure that what is said in a group session is confidential and that the safety of group members is never in jeopardy. Ideally, confidentiality must be maintained by an entire group of people who all understand the meaning of confidentiality. However, the counselor is not in control of violations of confidentiality because the counselor cannot control what is said outside of the group. In individual counseling, the counselor can guarantee confidentiality because the counselor is the only person who can break the confidentiality. The same is true with safety. The counselor cannot control what other members of the group do to each other either in the group or out of the group.

The group counselor must be trained as a group counselor. One area of training is in the use of counseling responses, which requires adequate experiential supervision in addition to didactic learning. The ASGW (1991) *Professional Standards for the Training of Group Workers* lists sixteen skills that are believed to be necessary for group counselors. They are listed in Table 4 (page 16) with the corresponding BCRG counseling responses.

Co-counseling in Groups

Two groups on the videocassette, CD-ROM, and Web site are co-counseled, as are many groups. Co-counseling is an effective way to train new group counselors and a way to provide support for experienced group counselors. Co-counseling is a collaborative effort that requires mutual respect and a willingness to work as a team. Gladding (1999, pp. 89–91) lists both the advantages and limitations of co-counseling:

Advantages	*Limitations*
Ease of handling the group in difficult situations	Lack of coordinated efforts
Uses of modeling	Too leader-focused
Feedback	Competition
Shared specialized knowledge	Collusion
Pragmatic considerations (coverage)	

ATTENDING and GIVING FEEDBACK are two responses used frequently in a co-counseled group. Both counselors can be doubly aware of what is happening in the group and give feedback to what they see and hear. However, complications can arise from being doubly aware. For example, one counselor might follow another counselor's response with the idea of strengthening the original response. This could be overwhelming to the group and often minimizes the original response. Co-counselors also may be tempted to explain what the other counselor has said or to "rescue" the other counselor. While there are exceptions, co-counselors should generally work in concert, not getting in each other's way. Co-counselors should avoid stacking their responses; that is, one counselor should wait for clients to respond to the other counselor before making an additional response.

To avoid the limitations of co-counseling and enhance the advantages, co-counselors should meet both before and after a group session to debrief and plan their roles. The dynamics of the group and options to responding should also be discussed. In addition, consultation with a third party may be helpful.

TABLE 4: ASGW COMPETENCIES AND BCRG COUNSELING RESPONSES

ASGW	BCRG
Encourage participation of group members	DIRECTING, GIVING FEEDBACK ALLOWING SILENCE
Observe and identify group process events	ATTENDING, GIVING FEEDBACK, PARAPHRASING
Attend to and acknowledge group member behavior	ATTENDING, GIVING FEEDBACK, PARAPHRASING
Clarify and summarize group member statements	CLARIFYING, PARAPHRASING
Open and close group sessions	OPENING OR CLOSING
Impart information in the group when necessary	Though not a counseling response, this may be a necessary task of the group counselor.
Model effective group leader behavior	Though not a counseling response, a very necessary function the group counselor.
Engage in appropriate self-disclosure in the group	SELF-DISCLOSING
Give and receive feedback in the group	GIVING FEEDBACK
Ask open ended questions in the group	QUESTIONING
Empathize with group members	EMPATHIZING
Confront group members behaviors	NOTING DISCREPANCY, NOTING A THEME, REFRAMING. NOTING A CONNECTION, PLAYING A HUNCH
Help group members attribute meaning to the experience	QUESTIONING, NOTING A THEME, NOTING A CONNECTION, PLAYING A HUNCH
Help group members integrate and apply learning	QUESTIONING, NOTING A THEME, NOTING A CONNECTION, PLAYING A HUNCH
Demonstrate ASGW ethical and professional standards of group practice	Though not a counseling response, a very necessary function of the group counselor.
Keep group on task in accomplishing goals	DIRECTING

Client Responses

What clients say in a group may be more important than the counselor's response. Research supports this premise. Quoting Yalom (1995):

> Considerable research emphasizes the importance many members place on working through relationships with other members rather than with the leader. To take one example, a team of researchers asked members, in a twelve-month follow-up of a short-term crisis group, to indicate the source of the help each had received. Forty-two percent felt that the group members and not the therapist had been helpful and 28 percent felt that both had been of aid. Only 5 percent stated that the therapist alone was a major contributor to change. The corpus of research has important implications for the technique of the group therapist: rather than focusing exclusively on the patient-therapist relationship, therapists must facilitate the development and working-through of interactions among members (pp. 44–45).

To test the premise of the research Yalom (1995) cited, the members of the groups in the BCRG videocassette and CD-ROM were asked the following three questions four months after the groups were taped:

1. What was the most meaningful thing that you heard in the group session?
2. Who said it?
3. Do you have any other feedback about the group experience?

Out of the 38 total client participants, 23 individuals were reached and responded. The results of this follow-up are in Appendix A. This data indicates that an overwhelming majority of clients, 21 out of 23 (91 percent), report that the most meaningful things they remember were comments made by other clients or interactions with other clients. This supports Yalom's (1995) belief that ". . . the real core of the therapeutic process in these therapy groups is an affectively charged, self-reflective, interpersonal interaction (p. 79)." What the counselor says is much less significant, as was stated by Aaron, Group 3/graduates, when he reflected on what was most meaningful to him. He remembered what another group member said: "I don't think it matters what the group counselors think." (See Amy, Group 3/graduates, 3.24.)

Comments made by members of the adolescent boys group support Yalom's (1995) therapeutic factor of universality. What seemed to be most meaningful to them was knowing that they were not alone. For example, Wallace states, "Even though I hang out with those guys, it was great to hear what they've been through. It's great to know somebody else out there knows what I've gone through. Other people can understand where I'm coming from." In addition, Mitchell's comment supports another therapeutic factor, group cohesion (Yalom, 1995), "It helped me understand where people are coming from. Like one of the guys I live with—he never said anything like that before. It helped me understand why people do the things they do."

Clients may make counseling responses with or without being asked or directed to do so by the counselor. Either phenomena can only happen in a group counseling setting. Clients are almost always ATTENDING, and, often with encouragement, SELF-DISCLOSING. Clients also make other significant responses. For example, midway in the development of Group 2/boys, James is QUESTIONING to challenge group experience (2.106): "You think it feels any different, then, if they had six other kids come in here that weren't in the system? Do you think we'd be talking about other, different stuff?" Not only do these questions challenge the group to look at themselves in the group and outside the group, but by saying "we'd be talking" he acknowledges his perception of the "we-ness" of the group.

The counselor can use DIRECTING or QUESTIONING to encourage a client to make a counseling response. For example, at (4.63), the counselor asks Kyle to tell Liz, after she has self-disclosed, how he sees her in the group. Kyle, thus, is SELF-DISCLOSING to acknowledge individual feeling in context: "It doesn't make me feel any different about you than I did already." In Group 5/adults, at (5.103), Counselor A asks I-Wei to use the response of QUESTIONING; Counselor A: "Could you ask her?" I-Wei: "What are you feeling right now?"

Counselors model their counseling responses and clients pick up on these and use them with each other; clients then respond to each others' counseling responses. At (2.330) and (2.334), the counselor asks James how he feels about her interrupting, but does not get a response. When Thomas (2.341) says, "How do you feel about her jumping in front of you like that?" (QUESTIONING to explore individual feeling in context), James responds. This process fosters the belief that it is the interpersonal interaction that is a significant source of therapeutic change for the client. Yalom (1995), noting research on the various therapeutic factors of group, says, "overall, however, the preponderance of research indicates that the power of the interactional outpatient group emanates from its interpersonal properties" (p. 105).

Clients responding to each other using therapeutic language may also be an example of group cohesiveness; that is, "the patient's relationship not only to the group therapist but to the group members and to the group as a whole" (Yalom, 1995, p. 48). At (1b.52), Lynn says, "Wow, in the first group we had I felt so naked. And now, I really feel more a sense of connection with the group and even as we're talking about struggles within, I'm hearing us talk about, I don't feel so separate, I feel part of the group. And a lot of the areas that I feel alone, I don't feel so alone." In this one response, the client not only acknowledges the sense of cohesiveness that she feels in the group, but she also is SELF-DISCLOSING and PARAPHRASING. Client responses may also be an example of imitative behavior (identification): "patients begin to approach problems by considering, not necessarily on a conscious level, what some other members or the therapist would think or do in the same situation" (Yalom, 1995, p. 85). Another example of a client responding to other group members is made by Matt at (5.79). He acknowledges what he sees others getting out of the group by PARAPHRASING and NOTING A DISCREPENCY: "And it sounds like you are actually getting something out of this despite what you said earlier that you weren't."

Other examples of client-generated counseling responses are:

REFRAMING: Linda (1a.68), "Maybe your using the term *selfish* comes across to me in many ways like guilt, I'm going to talk about that. Guilt that . . . "

QUESTIONING: Jean (1a.79), "I, I just want to know from Lynn, how would it be if we end right now?"

EMPATHIZING: Dorothy (1b.53), ". . . I know that even in this group we've tenderly gone, well not tenderly, but gingerly gone there and, um, that's a hard thing to do, without getting angry."

PLAYING A HUNCH: Aaron (3.17), "I almost feel like it's uncomfortable for the counselors and that you're doing something that you feel uncomfortable with being in the group."

NOTING A DISCREPENCY: Barbara (1a.74),"You know, you keep saying, you keep saying weird, but you keep talking about it."

DIRECTING: Eric (2.22), "Let's talk about something beside sports or video games."

NOTING A CONNECTION: Kyle (4.62), "That's why some people are afraid to share their feelings because the people might look at them different and have different opinions about them than what you want."

To determine the extent of counseling responses made by clients without direction, the unedited tapes of the eight sessions filmed for the CD-ROM and videocassette were examined to determine the number of times that clients used counseling responses. Determining client-generated counseling responses was done with the understanding that the raters, while following the definitions in this worktext, are ultimately using their own judgement to determine whether a response is, or could be, a counseling response. As noted above in the discussion of using the pronoun "I," many client-generated counseling responses start with "I" and include more self-disclosure, unlike most counselor responses. For example, Vee says (1a.28), "As I sit here and listened to you, Dorothy, I kind of made a switch. I know I would be concerned if it were mine. But, for a moment I was transported to, uh, my mother's shoes, and the choices her son made, my brother. I am just sitting here feeling somewhat of your grief. Thank you for saying what you said because that, that's helped me." A counselor, EMPATHIZING, acknowledging Dorothy's grief, might simply say, "You're feeling your grief now." Note also that Vee's response also acknowledges the impact of one group member's disclosure on another. ATTENDING is very difficult to measure in a group from a tape, but obvious attending behavior (actively nodding and verbal "uh-huh"s were counted. SELF-DISCLOSING was counted only when it referenced the context of the group, since so many client responses are self-disclosing their own story, but not necessarily as a group counseling response. OPENING OR CLOSING and ALLOWING SILENCE, as used by clients, are responses that were not evidenced in the sessions. Intents and focuses are not charted, though it was noted that the focus on the group increased in every group. The counseling intents were not surmised.

The results of tallying the frequency of client-generated counseling responses at ten-minute intervals in the unedited tapes are charted in Appendix A, Chart 6. Adding the total of all groups showed that the frequency increased with time, leveling off near the end. This increase in client-generated counseling responses may be an example of "interpersonal output" identified in the findings by Butler and Furriman, cited by Yalom (1995): "The therapeutic factors of cohesiveness, self-understanding, and interpersonal output were more valued by patients the longer they participated in the group" (p. 102). Group 3/graduates, Group 4/students, and Group 5/adults showed a similar pattern. Group 2/boys did not follow this pattern; the frequency of client-generated counseling responses actually decreased in the middle of the session. However, the frequency of client-generated counseling responses was consistently higher in this group of adolescent boys than in any other group. The inconsistency may be because, developmentally, adolescents are not as consistent in their group behavior. The higher frequency of counseling responses may be a result of them being less inhibited in GIVING FEEDBACK, are maybe more aware of what is happening in the group and more willing to say so by PARAPHRASING, and are more likely to NOTE A DISCREPENCY by challenging each other. Another hypothesis is that they became more cohesive and the use of counseling responses is an example of this cohesiveness.

Nonverbal Responses

ATTENDING and ALLOWING SILENCE are clearly nonverbal counseling responses. Other counseling responses can be made nonverbally. For example, after a group has met several times, the counselor may open by a simple gesture of opening the hands; an inquisitive look may imply a question and the need for clarification; and a pointing finger may be directive. In a group, where there may be many interpretations of nonverbal behavior, the voice inflection, gestures, posture, and facial expressions of the counselor may enhance or distract from the counseling response.

Noncounseling Responses

Group counselors make verbal and nonverbal responses in a group that are important for the betterment of the group, but are not considered counseling responses. These responses may be outside the role of counselor; for example, the counselor may need to assume the role of teacher. The following are counseling tasks or counselor behaviors that are outside the definition of making a counseling response:

1. The group counselor models how to respond appropriately in a group whether it be asking a question or respecting personal differences. Modeling is an important part of what the counselor does or how the counselor acts, but is not necessarily a response to what is happening in the group. However, any response or behavior, counseling or not, could be considered modeling.
2. Evaluating and diagnosing are tasks the counselor may need to accomplish while in the group, but not as a direct response to the group. Counseling responses, especially questioning, can be made as part of an evaluation or diagnostic process. Evaluating or diagnosing may be the primary tasks of screening for a group.
3. Group exercises can be a valuable part of the group experience for clients, but as with giving information or suggestions, the use of exercises is more of a counseling task than a response. Yet directing, as a counseling response, is often what the counselor does to accomplish part of an exercise.
4. The counselor may find it necessary to impart information, give suggestions, or correct misinformation for the benefit of part or all of the group. Establishing norms and explaining confidentiality are good examples. The group counselor will also need to get information from clients necessary for the functioning of the group.
5. The counselor may choose to focus on a specific topic, especially in a curriculum-based group. While this may be valuable for the group, it is not a counseling response because the focus is on a topic rather than the group or any member of the group.
6. The group counselor may also have the responsibility for the physical and temporal needs of the group, which may be more demanding than for an individual. The group counselor must determine the size of the group and the frequency of sessions.
7. If norms are broken and the consequences are not enforced by the group, the counselor may find it necessary to act as disciplinarian.

Timing of Responses

Various authors who have created models of group counseling offer suggestions of tasks and interventions to be offered at different stages of development. However, variables of the group experience are too complex to be able to say, "Use this counseling response at this time." In individual counseling, counselors initially withhold directive and interpretive responses, and do not self-disclose until a relationship has been established with the client. But in group counseling, the counselor may need to be more directive early on to facilitate the interaction among members or to establish and reinforce norms; the group counselor may also need to self-disclose and give feedback to model for group members.

While the fifteen basic counseling responses and combination responses can be made at any time in the life of a group, group counselors must always consider what counseling response seems most appropriate to what is happening or what might happen in the group. With practice and supervision, just as in individual counseling, the group counselor can develop timing that reflects both the style of the counselor and the culture of the group.

Responding to the Difficult Client

The difficult client is more of a concern in a group because of the influence on other group members and the dynamic of the group itself. Almost every text on group counseling includes a section on the difficult client. Every teacher and group counselor knows that almost every group has a member that is in (or possibly chooses) the difficult role. Kottler (1994) says,

> There appears to be an unwritten law of the universe that for every conglomeration of persons numbering more than a few who are gathered together for a common purpose under a set of rules, there will always be one person, although well meaning and good natured, will have quite inappropriate behavior and responses (p. 173).

There will be group members who are not "well meaning and good natured." There are some people that are not appropriate for a group. Careful screening might prevent inappropriate individuals from becoming the difficult client by excluding them from the group. Of course, the nature of the group will determine the screening criteria. The dilemma is that the difficult client may need the group the most. And, if people play the same role in a group as they play outside the group, it can be expected that the difficult client is difficult in other situations. The group may help this person change their out-of-group behavior as well. The counselor must determine the criteria for group membership, understanding that there is not an ideal client, as well as determine the criteria for discontinuing membership if a member's behavior is beyond the established norms of the group.

Descriptions of and strategies to deal with difficult clients are offered by Kottler (1994) and Yalom (1995) among others. Clients are described by their behaviors, such as silent, monopolizing, boring, and complaining. Resistance to the group process is a common characteristic of the difficult client. The client that challenges the counselor or scapegoats other clients is also noted by most authors as possibly problematic. Breaking of norms, conflict among members, and challenging the counselor are not uncommon experiences; they might be considered problematic only if they represent a pattern of behavior in a group that the counselor wants to change.

Unless serious interventions are needed, consider following the counseling intents, when encountering the client who is having difficulty being part of the group:

- To acknowledge

  In response to the silent client, "I notice that you haven't said anything in group today."

  GIVING FEEDBACK *to acknowledge* individual behavior in context

  In response to several members of the of group scapegoating one member, "I notice that several of you are blaming Mary for what is happening."

  GIVING FEEDBACK *to acknowledge* subgroup behavior

  Group members need to first be aware of their behavior because they may not be aware their behavior is inappropriate. Once they become aware, their behavior may change.

- To explore

  In response to the resistant client, "Tell the group more about how the two of you are feeling about being in the group."

  CLARIFYING *to explore* subgroup feeling in context

Difficult clients may need to explore the etiology of their difficulty. This may elicit responses from other members of the group. This exploration may change the behavior.

In response to the group challenging the group counselor (which may or may not be difficult behavior), "Talk more about how it is for the group to not have me responding the way you want me to."

CLARIFYING *to explore* group experience

- To challenge

In response to disruptive behavior, "What other ways might the group respond when the group disagrees with a member of this group?"

QUESTIONING *to challenge* group behavior

In response to the group breaking a group norm (which may or may not be difficult behavior), "How is it for the group when other members use language that the group decided not to use in the group?"

QUESTIONING *to challenge* subgroup experience

To challenge the client to change their behavior in the group and reflect on how the group behavior may be characteristic of behavior outside the group is never easy, but can result in significant in-group and out-of-group change.

Note that in dealing with the difficult client, behavior is most frequently the focus of the counselor's attention, though the focus of the counseling response may not be, as in the previous explore examples. Seldom do experiences, feelings or thoughts provoke the counselor to label the client as difficult. In fact, the self-disclosing of experience, thoughts, and feelings often helps the group members (and the counselor) better understand the client's behavior. Also, seldom does the group counselor need to cope with difficult *group* behavior or difficult *subgroup* behavior. If that occurs, the same counseling responses can be used with a different focus.

The counselor can *use the group* to deal with difficult behavior. For example:

"How does the group feel when John interrupts?"

QUESTIONING to challenge group feeling

"I'd like the group to give Sue some feedback about how they feel when she does most of the talking in group."

DIRECTING to challenge group behavior in context

The counselor can then follow with, the "one-two punch" (see page 43). For example:

"How was it for you to get this feedback from the group?"

and

"How was it for the group to give this feedback?"

QUESTIONING to challenge individual experience

QUESTIONING to challenge group experience

While *difficult* is a familiar term, the reader might consider *reframing* the labeling of client from "difficult client" to "a client with difficult behavior" or "a challenge for the counselor" or "an opportunity for the group." The difficult client for one counselor (or group) may be the interesting client or a learning resource for another. It might also be important for the rest of the group to have a difficult member within the group; it might help the members cope with a difficult person and develop skills that could be transferable outside the group.

1.1	Counselor	"Where would the group like to start?" ■ OPENING ● to acknowledge ▼ group experience *Note the opening response is in question form.*

Format for Examples, Exercises, and Transcripts

In the transcripts, each client and counselor response is consecutively numbered. The numbers correspond to the videocassette, CD-ROM video sessions, and the CD-ROM. The first number is the group number, followed by a lowercase letter if there are multiple sessions (1b.5). This group number is followed by the number of the client or counselor response (3.14). Multiple counselor responses are differentiated by small case letters (2.300a and 2.300b). Groups are identified by number and name at the top of each transcript. The respective speaker and the verbatim transcript follow in quotes. On the next line, the identified RESPONSE, intent, and focus will be preceded by the square, circle, and triangle icons, respectively. (This is also true throughout the worktext.) Any comments will be in *italics*.

In the worktext exercises for the videocassette, transcripts used for the exercises will not have the bold identifications for the selected interactions. Students make these themselves as part of the exercises and then compare their identifications with the SUGGESTED IDENTIFICATIONS that are also included with each exercise. In the transcripts for Groups 1 and 2, a CD-ROM icon with an up-arrow ⬆ is used at the beginning of clips, and a CD-ROM icon with a down-arrow ⬇ is used at the end of clips. In the identification of counseling responses, the intents use the language "to acknowledge," "to explore," or "to challenge"; the additives of context and immediacy, use the language *in context* and *with immediacy*.

Throughout this worktext, the CD-ROM, and the videocassette, the rectangle icon denotes responses, the circle denotes intents, and the triangle denotes focus. See the rectangle, circle, and triangle graphics in Figures 1, 2, and 3, respectively, Appendix A.

Limitations

This learning package focuses on how the counselor responds in a counseling group. Its purpose is limited to presenting counseling responses in groups in a simplified training format. The responses in this text, the CD-ROM, and the videocassette are basic to any group counseling interaction, at any stage of the counseling process, and are expected to be supplemented in counselor training programs with theoretical strategies and interventions relative to specific types of groups or specific group populations. This package does not attempt to compare or compete with the definitive works of Irwin Yalom and others. Yalom's *The Theory and Practice of Group Psychotherapy* (1995), for example, is invaluable in its theoretical delineation and research-supported explanations of group process, the therapists role in fostering group cohesion, and the therapeutic factors of the group experience. Gerald Corey (2000), Samuel Gladding (1999), and Jeffrey Kottler (1994) offer extensive works on group development, the tasks and responsibilities of the group counselor and group counseling ethics, that should be a part of every group counseling curriculum.

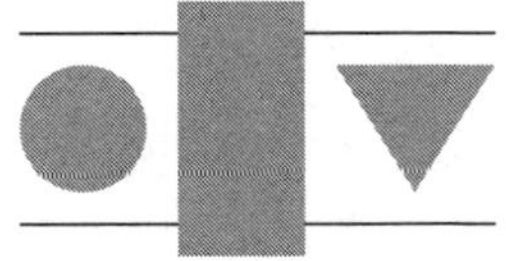

PART 2
Descriptions and Examples

In this part, the fifteen basic counseling responses are described and exemplified. The responses are divided into five descriptive categories: essential, passive, active, interpretive, and discretionary. These are the same fifteen counseling responses named in *Basic Counseling Responses* (1999), supporting the belief that counseling responses are generic and foundational to individual and group counseling. However, variables that distinguish group versus individual responses will be discussed and group specific examples given. The fifteen descriptions will be divided into three parts per response:

- An edited version of the counseling response description from *Basic Counseling Responses* (1999).
- A discussion of the group applicability of the response.
- An example or examples of the respective response used in a group. Intents and focuses are identified and comments made when appropriate.

The focus of the response is the significant difference between a counseling response given to an individual versus a counseling response given to a group or part of a group. At the same time, the actual response, whether it be PARAPHRASING or SELF-DISCLOSING is the same in either situation. What is different, in addition to the focus, is how and when the particular response is used. For example, in the description of QUESTIONING, the "one-two punch" is actually two QUESTIONING responses used together and is unique to the group counseling situation. The one-two punch is unique to group counseling clients because one question is focused on the individual, and the other on the group.

Choosing what response to use and when to use it is part of the group counselor's role. One factor that influences that decision is the intent of the group counselor to encourage clients to respond to each other, as noted by Yalom (1995):

> In the individual format, the therapist functions as the sole designated direct change agent. The group therapist functions far more indirectly. In other words, if it is the group members who,

> in their interaction, set into motion the many therapeutic factors, then it is the group therapist's task to create a group culture maximally conducive to effective group interaction (p. 109–110).

The essential responses of OPENING OR CLOSING and ATTENDING are the most generic of all counseling responses. OPENING OR CLOSING happens *only at the beginning or end*, during group and individual sessions and ATTENDING is *continuous* in both venues.

The *passive* responses, GIVING FEEDBACK, PARAPHRASING, and EMPATHIZING, are given by the counselor without expectation of an active or obvious response from group clients. The responses are given to show that the counselor is aware of what an individual, part of the group, or the group as a whole is saying (PARAPHRASING), doing (GIVING FEEDBACK), and feeling (EMPATHIZING). EMPATHIZING and GIVING FEEDBACK are commonly used by clients, whether or not directed to do so. In a group situation these responses are given by the counselor to *model* appropriate ways for clients to respond to each other.

The *active* responses of CLARIFYING, DIRECTING, and QUESTIONING are given by the counselor to facilitate group interaction, with the expectation that one or more clients in the group will respond with:

- More concrete information or examples;
- Specific requests of the counselor; or
- Answers to the counselor's questions. (If clients respond directly to the counselor; the counselor may want to re-direct or re-question the group.)

DIRECTING and CLARIFYING are sometimes phrased as a question. DIRECTING and QUESTIONING are often used in group counseling and are especially useful when encouraging members of a group to respond to other group members. These are often requests to the group to make *passive* responses, such as, "Could the group be GIVING FEEDBACK to each other about how you see each other coming across in the group?" (DIRECTING to challenge group behavior in context *in question form*).

Clients often ask questions of each other, though the intention may be to get information rather than to explore or challenge. Questions may also be for clarification, but they are often for the clarification of the asker, rather than as a counseling response that asks for clarification to benefit the client. If the counselor senses that what a client is saying is not clear to the group, the counselor may say, "Tell the group more about that" (CLARIFYING to explore individual experience). This response is for the benefit of the group and for the clarification of the individual.

In group counseling, there are many opportunities for the counselor to use active responses since, once again, a distinguishing task of the group counselor is to encourage group interaction.

The *interpretive* responses—PLAYING A HUNCH, NOTING A THEME, NOTING A DISCREPANCY, NOTING A CONNECTION, and REFRAMING—are also used in groups. However, because they are interpretations emanating from the counselor, they may not be especially different from individual counseling, other than in their focus and frequency. There are more incidences for NOTING A DISCREPENCY in a group because there is a *greater* frequency of differing responses form a larger number (more than one) of clients.

NOTING A CONNECTION and NOTING A THEME, however, require the counselor to look for commonalities within the group as a whole, much like the counselor would do with an individual. The opportunities to do this may be *less* in a group, because of the diversity of the members. PLAYING A HUNCH and REFRAMING are similar in this regard. It may be difficult to find a common theme, especially in the early stages of a group, and even more difficult to reframe for an entire group. Group counselors may find more opportunities for PLAYING A HUNCH or REFRAMING with individuals in the group or a subgroup, rather than the group as a whole.

Therefore, interpretive responses may be similar in both individual and group counseling with one significant exception: When the counselor shares an interpretation, or when an interpretation is seen as confrontational, the counselor models ways for the group members to respond to each other. Therefore, the counselor must respond with respect, possibly with tentativeness, and certainly with the caveat that they are interpretations or possibilities. It will take some familiarity with the group dynamics before the counselor may offer an interpretation that would:

- Suggest different possibilities (REFRAMING);
- Give the counselor's view of the relationships between thoughts, behaviors, and feelings (NOTING A CONNECTION, NOTING A THEME, NOTING A DISCREPENCY); or
- Give the counselor's internal frame of reference (PLAYING A HUNCH).

Unlike other responses, interpretive responses often overlap because of their speculative nature; the counselor may have a hunch that there is a connection. Also, interpretive responses are generally not delivered as a question, though they may be given with some tentativeness. And again, interpretive responses may in many cases seem to be challenging or confrontational for the individual or the group.

The *discretionary* responses of ALLOWING SILENCE and SELF-DISCLOSING are curiously unique in a group. Silence is less likely to happen because there are more people to break the silence. Though the counselor may be ALLOWING SILENCE, members of the group will often choose to interrupt the silence, making the identification of this response difficult. Thus, the impact of silence, that is the chance for internal reflection, is less likely in a group. The opposite effect is true of self-disclosure. Self-disclosure from group members is necessary and constant. Counselor SELF-DISCLOSING may be necessary to set a norm for the group that it is safe, necessary, and appropriate to self-disclose. ("I know that I am nervous, as a counselor, the first night of group." (SELF-DISCLOSING to acknowledge group feeling). As a counseling response, SELF-DISCLOSING should be given with caution because it can risk taking the focus off the group. Self-disclosure is consistently done by clients, and responded to by clients, so it is even more discretionary in its use.

Appendix A, Table 1 compares *BCRG* to responses and skills of other group counseling models.

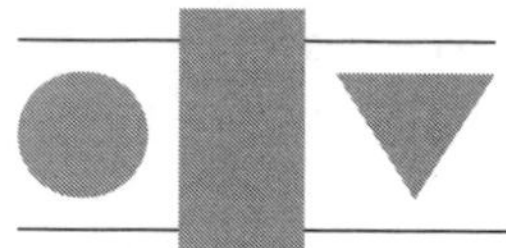

OPENING OR CLOSING

TYPE OF RESPONSE
ESSENTIAL

OPENING OR CLOSING a counseling session is not necessarily considered therapeutic, per se, but may be very important to the entire process and relationship. Openings set the tone and momentum, closings provide closure. Different situations require that different information be given to clients in the first session. Generally, clients need to know the qualifications of the counselor, times, dates and costs, as well as confidentiality parameters. Clients may also need an explanation about the counseling process.

The opening of a counseling session can be awkward for both clients and counselor. Clients are understandably cautious about sharing their lives with a new person. Tension and anxiety are a natural response to new situations; thus resistance is very common. Counselors are encouraged to be very patient, especially in the initial session. Reducing the initial tension may not necessarily be the goal of the counselor. The counselor needs to decide what his/her views are regarding the optimal level of anxiety. It is generally agreed upon that giving some structure to the initial session helps the client(s) feel safe and promotes trust. Giving clients initial choices can reduce the anxiety: "Where would you like to sit?"

It is generally assumed to be the counselor's responsibility to decide when the session begins (after the clients sit down, for example, rather than in the hall walking to the office). A common phrase for a counselor to start a session is, "Where would you like to start?" This phrase puts the choice and responsibility on the clients.

Counselors can assume the responsibility for closing a session, though this, too, can be given to the clients. Some counselors use clocks or hourglasses and let the clients know that it is their responsibility to pace themselves and end the session on time. Ending on time is almost always essential given time constraints of both counselor and clients; plus many theorists believe that it is important for clients to learn to work in a specific time frame. A common phrase is, "We have five minutes left. How would you like to close?" OPENING OR CLOSING can be in question or statement form.

The ending of the counseling relationship is also important because it may mirror the ending of other relationships. Counselors should allow ample time to process the ending of this relationship and can use questions to challenge as closing responses: "How has our time together been for you?" or "How is it to end our relationship?"

Generally, the intent of opening is to explore what the client(s) may want to discuss. The intent of closing is generally to acknowledge the end of a session. OPENING OR CLOSING responses may focus on experience, feeling, thought, and/or behavior. Since most responses of this type are open-ended to allow the client(s) to chose the specific focus, the focus is *primarily* on experience. Although OPENING OR CLOSING refers to the immediate situation, it is not an immediacy focus unless the counselor adds a specific immediacy focus, such as, "How is it to end at this moment?"

OPENING OR CLOSING in Groups

Especially in a group, OPENING OR CLOSING can be simply stating a fact (see the following examples 2 and 4). Therefore, they are identified by their *placement* rather than their content. Several suggestions from Corey (2000) show how other counseling responses are used to open:

> 1) Participants can be asked to briefly state what they want to get from the session . . . 2) It is useful to give people a chance to express any thoughts that they may have had about the previous session or to bring up for consideration any unresolved issues from a previous session . . . 3) Participants may be asked to report on the progress or difficulties they experienced during the week . . . 4) The group leader may want to make some observations about the previous meeting or relate some thoughts that have occurred to him or her since the group met last (p. 52).

Suggestions 1 and 3 above are QUESTIONING to open ("What would you like to get from the group today?"; "How have you progressed with what we talked about last week?") Suggestion 2 can be QUESTIONING or DIRECTING ("Any unresolved issues to bring to the group?" or "Share with the group any thoughts from last week"). Suggestion 4 can be SELF-DISCLOSING or PLAYING A HUNCH ("I felt uncomfortable after we closed the last session." "It seemed like some people left the group angry last session.")

Some counselors prefer to open groups with specific group exercises so members can become more comfortable with each other. For example, each member can pair off with another member and get to know each other's likes and dislikes. Then the pairs rejoin as a group and introduce each other to the entire group. However, it is our belief that the "power of groups" will occur as the group continues and individuals naturally share their experiences, thoughts, feelings, and behaviors with each other. Choosing to use exercises is an option based on one's own preference.

When CLOSING, it is not necessary to have all issues resolved between group members. These unresolved issues can be addressed in the next session and may set the stage for a great deal of growth to take place between sessions. If it is the last session, it is important to spend time exploring any unresolved issues, what growth has taken place, and saying goodbye. Therefore, no new issues should be raised because there will not be a next session to address any issues that would arise.

Paralleling the suggestion that the opening responsibility and focus be put on the group, the counselor can also say, "How would the group like to end today?" or "We have discussed anger and guilt today; how was it for the group to talk about these issues?" Asking the group to reflect on the experience of the group is a way of applying the self-reflective loop (Yalom, 1995). PARAPHRASING (or a longer summary) is another common response for ending a group.

CLOSING, whether it be a single session or for the life of the group, may provide the opportunity to reflect on other endings. Ample time should be provided to close, and the counselor may find it necessary to interrupt the flow of the group to meet the necessity of stopping on time. As a group progresses, the counselor may relinquish the responsibility to open and close a session or clients may assume that responsibility themselves.

EXAMPLES OF OPENING OR CLOSING IN GROUPS

1	Counselor	"Where would the group like to start?" ■ OPENING ● to explore ▼ group experience
2	Counselor	"It is time to get started." ■ OPENING ● to acknowledge ▼ group experience
3.1	Counselor	"Shall we get started?" ■ OPENING ● to acknowledge ▼ group experience
3.2	Client	"It's hard to get this group started."
4	Counselor	"We're going to need to stop right now." ■ CLOSING ● to acknowledge ▼ group experience

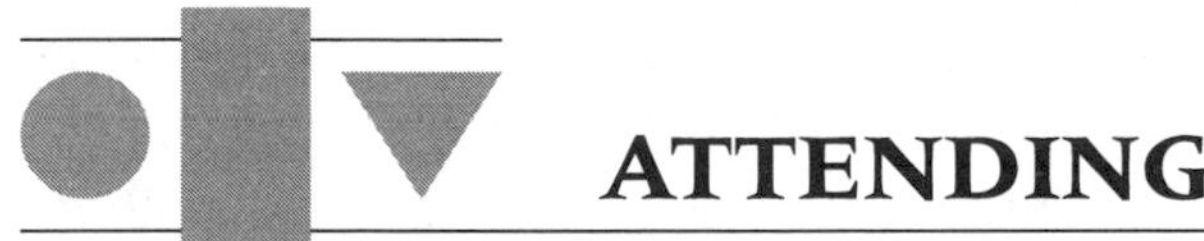

ATTENDING

TYPE OF RESPONSE
ESSENTIAL

ATTENDING means giving undivided attention to the client(s). It is the art of being with the client(s). It is also the art of paying attention to what you see and hear rather than what you know. Being attended to, being heard, helps the client(s) and encourages self-reflection.

It is important to give the client(s) plenty of time and space. Thus, part of ATTENDING is to slow the pace by resisting the temptation to talk or to keep the conversation moving. It is also important to allow for silences, again resisting the temptation to fill the voids of a conversation.

ATTENDING, like many things in counseling, is different from conversation in social or work situations. Counselors must refrain from learned behaviors such as talking about oneself and asking a lot of questions, to avoid lulls and silences. Thus, while ATTENDING may seem simple, it actually can be difficult as it requires that the counselor truly pay attention to what the client(s) is saying and doing, rather than what the counselor is thinking. ATTENDING is something that counselors do all the time with all clients and, thus, is an integral part of every other counseling response. ATTENDING is mostly nonverbal (that is, maintaining appropriate eye contact and an open posture), although an occasional "uh-huh" or "um-hmm" is uttered by the counselor. Being attentive also shows respect and compassion.

ATTENDING is usually intended to acknowledge the client(s). The counselor may focus on feelings, thoughts, or behaviors, but since this is a nonverbal response, the focus is usually on the experience of being with the client(s) in the present situation.

ATTENDING in Groups

The group counselor must always be aware of what is happening in the group verbally and nonverbally. The counselor must always be watching and listening. In a group this means watching and listening to several people, unlike individual counseling where one is attending to an individual.

ATTENDING may also provide the counselor with information to use when making other counseling responses. Attending by the counselor also models for the group members. Clients generally attend to each other. Nonattending behavior may need to be challenged by the counselor.

Jacobs, Masson, and Harvill (1998) use the term *scanning* to denote what the group counselor does:

> Leaders gather valuable information by scanning the group with their eyes . . . if the leader does what is natural, which would be to look exclusively at the person speaking, she misses information that is very helpful in facilitating the group . . . Most beginning leaders can learn rather quickly to scan the group while they are talking. However, learning to scan when someone else is talking takes practice (p. 123).

Scanning also encourages the clients to speak to one another rather than exclusively to the counselor. If a client is speaking to the counselor and the counselor begins to scan the group, the client will generally follow the example of the counselor and look to the group members for eye contact. When the group is co-counseled, it is customary for one counselor to scan the group while the other counselor is speaking. This way, important nonverbal information can be picked up by the observing counselor.

EXAMPLE OF ATTENDING IN GROUPS

1	COUNSELOR	Looking around the group, nodding as one client is talking, keeping eye contact with all clients. ■ ATTENDING ● to acknowledge ▼ group experience *The counselor is attending to the group experience in the broad sense; behavior, thoughts, and feelings are also attended to less specifically.*

EMPATHIZING, PARAPHRASING, GIVING FEEDBACK

TYPE OF RESPONSE
PASSIVE

Paraphrasing, summarizing, reflecting, reflection of feeling, reflection of content, mirroring, parroting, and empathizing are terms used by various counselor educators to denote counseling responses that let the client(s) know the counselor is listening and reflect what the counselor has seen or heard.

Generally PARAPHRASING and summarizing are ways of telling the client(s) what the counselor heard, in the counselor's own words. Summarizing is the same as PARAPHRASING, but generally covers more information, such as responses from the complete session, rather than one or two client responses. EMPATHIZING, or reflection of feelings, adds to the counselor's sense of what the client(s) is feeling. GIVING FEEDBACK is stating to the client(s) what the counselor observes. These responses each have a particular focus:

- EMPATHIZING is a response to feeling
- PARAPHRASING is a response to experience, thought, and/or behavior
- GIVING FEEDBACK is a response to *observed* behavior

An example of PARAPHRASING is: "You are saying . . . " or "What I hear you saying . . ." An example of EMPATHIZING is: "You feel . . . " A counselor GIVING FEEDBACK could say, "I notice tears in your eyes as you are talking" or "You have used the word *control* several times."

Generally, the intent of all three responses is to acknowledge, though naming the intent or the response can be ambiguous. For example, the counselor says, "I notice that you are smiling while you are talking about feeling sad." While this sounds like GIVING FEEDBACK to acknowledge client(s) behavior and EMPATHIZING to acknowledge feelings, the intent is most likely to challenge the discrepancy between the feelings and the observed behavior. Therefore, this is the response of NOTING A DISCREPANCY to challenge client feeling and client behavior.

EMPATHIZING requires that the counselor join with the client(s) and try to understand how it feels to be that individual, with all their unique qualities and perspectives. At the same time, it is important that the counselor remain separate from their experience. If this is done successfully, the client(s) will feel understood at a core level. This is a very different experience from what they might get from a friend. Usually a friend will say, "I know exactly how you feel," whereas a counselor responds, "You're feeling sad."

EMPATHIZING about client(s) feelings requires that the counselor have some understanding of his/her feelings even though the counselor may not have actually had the same feeling. The counselor may, in fact, *not* understand the feelings, or experience, or behavior. This is okay!

The important aspect of being empathetic is the *desire* to understand and communicating that desire. The counselor can always ask, "Am I understanding you correctly?" The counselor can check for understanding with the client(s) whether the counselor is understanding him/her. If not, then the client(s) can clarify his/her own understanding and at the same time know that the counselor cares enough to try to understand. This is one of the goals of counseling.

EMPATHIZING with client(s) feelings is also expressed nonverbally. A client(s) may be talking about a painful experience while clutching his/her throat. The counselor, by imitating the gesture, shows that the counselor understands the pain.

PARAPHRASING what the client(s) is telling the counselor is usually expressed in a sentence or two used throughout the session: "This is what I heard you saying . . . " or "You *are* telling me that . . . " The essential feature is to let the client(s) hear the essence of their statement. It is important to restate some of the client(s)' own words and add words of the counselor to help the client(s) know that the counselor truly hears what was said.

A longer paraphrase, also called a summary, can be used to the end a session or to transition to a new topic. For example, "You have been talking about your family, feelings at work, and your relationship with your girlfriend." PARAPHRASING differs from GIVING FEEDBACK in that GIVING FEEDBACK generally notes specific words or phrases that the client(s) has used that the counselor wants to highlight.

GIVING FEEDBACK regarding the clients verbal or non-verbal behavior is simply telling the client(s) what you see and hear while you are together: "I see that you are smiling"; "I heard your voice crack when you said "daughter"; "I notice that your arms have been crossed most of the session." In some contexts, outside of the counseling relationship, GIVING FEEDBACK is seen as Person A telling Person B what Person A thinks or feels about Person B. This may be in terms of personality characteristics, job performance, or test results. Guidelines to GIVING FEEDBACK in a counseling relationship include owning the feedback, being positive and specific, noting behavior not personal traits, and not putting the person receiving the feedback on the defensive. In this model, GIVING FEEDBACK is only the act of sharing precisely what the counselor has heard or observed.

Most often, the information given back to the client(s) is not new to the client(s). Sometimes, because of the focus of attention on the statement or behavior, the information may feel new, thus increasing the client's self-awareness. Receiving feedback may be threatening or the person may not see the feedback as increasing self-awareness. Therefore, it may be important to follow-up with, "How was it for you to get this feedback?" (QUESTIONING to challenge with the focus on the experience plus immediacy.)

GIVING FEEDBACK about specific observed behavior is different from PARAPHRASING about the client's feelings or experiences of the client(s) in that the counselor is reiterating a specific observation, rather than encapsulating, using the counselor's wording, what has been said by the client(s).

EMPATHIZING in Groups

Most group counselors do not use the response EMPATHIZING frequently. This is quite different from individual counseling where a large portion of responses are empathic. The difference is that in a group setting it is more therapeutic for the other members of the group rather than the counselor to express empathy. When other members in the group can express empathy—share that they too have had similar experiences—cohesion is enhanced. The advantage a group has over individual counseling is there are more individuals in the room who can show their empathy and therefore help the individual feel more understood. To create this atmosphere in the group it is important that the counselor initially model empathy. Later in the group the counselor will use QUESTIONING to elicit empathic responses from the client(s); for example, "How does the group feel when they hear Bill talk about his situation?"

EMPATHIZING often is accompanied by a softer voice, or leaning forward to imply deeper understanding. Carroll and Wiggins (1997) speak to the "art" of being empathic in a group:

> To remain distant, to orchestrate the process yet be present psychologically, and to communicate with empathy to a given member in moments of joy and pain is an art (p. 59).

EXAMPLES OF EMPATHIZING IN GROUPS

1	COUNSELOR	"There is a sadness in the group right now." ■ EMPATHIZING ● to acknowledge ▼ group feeling with immediacy in context
2	COUNSELOR	"You know, I kind of feel this, low, sort of energy in the room, almost some sadness." ■ EMPATHIZING ● to acknowledge ▼ group feeling
3	COUNSELOR	"Several members of the group are angry with each other." ■ EMPATHIZING ● to acknowledge ▼ subgroup feeling

PARAPHRASING in Groups

PARAPHRASING is often done by the counselor to help the group see what is happening in the group from an unbiased perspective. It can change the pace of the session, slow down a very hectic interchange, or bring the focus back to an important issue that is getting lost in the session. When the focus is on the group or the sub-group, a paraphrase can help members hear what is said by others, rather than just focusing on what the individual is saying.

PARAPHRASING is often stated as a question. This is not paraphrasing per se, but is often meant to be. When this is done, PARAPHRASING becomes an active response because the listener may feel a need to answer the question. In non-question form, it is passive because it does not anticipate an answer. PARAPHRASING in question form may be seen as a way the counselor confirms what is said by the individual or group. Using the term summarizing rather than paraphrasing, Jacobs, Masson, and Harvill (1998) state:

"The skill of summarizing is a must for all group leaders. Groups often generate material from a wide range of viewpoints. Because members are busy listening and sharing during the session, they often do not pick up on or remember many of the details. Therefore, thoughtful and concise summaries are helpful to group members" (p. 116).

EXAMPLES OF PARAPHRASING IN GROUPS

1	COUNSELOR	"So some members of the group are saying that it is difficult when people disagree with each other." ■ PARAPHRASING ● to acknowledge ▼ subgroup experience
2	COUNSELOR	"The group has agreed to keep all the information confidential." ■ PARAPHRASING ● to acknowledge ▼ group experience *This could be group behavior or possibly thought*
3.1	CLIENT A	"I don't like to be asked a lot of personal questions if I am not ready. I don't want to get mad and yell at you guys."
3.2	CLIENT B	"I feel the same way. I need for people to respect me and not push me."
3.3	COUNSELOR	"It sounds like for you two to feel safe in the group, people need to respect your space and not push." ■ PARAPHRASING ● to acknowledge ▼ subgroup feeling in context *Note that this is a paraphrase of more than one person*
3.4	CLIENT C	"Yeah (laughs). Don't worry, I won't start any fights. I'll try not to anyway (laughs)."

GIVING FEEDBACK in Groups

GIVING FEEDBACK in a group is a very significant therapeutic response, especially when the feedback is given by other members of the group, rather than the counselor. Therefore, it is likely that the counselor will give less direct feedback to the group, but will ask other group members to give feedback to the whole group, a sub-group, or an individual. For example, the counselor might use the response of QUESTIONING to encourage the group to give feedback to an individual member: "How is Sally's behavior in the group affecting others?" Kottler (1995) notes the importance of GIVING FEEDBACK in groups:

> The use of feedback in group is limitless. It is one of the best services provided throughout the sessions and various therapeutic stages because it is so rare to get helpful, honest feedback in the real world (p. 80).
>
> A skilled group leader gives specific and honest feedback based on his or her observation of and reaction to the members' behaviors and encourages the members to give feedback to one another (Corey, p. 42).

EXAMPLES OF GIVING FEEDBACK IN GROUPS

1	COUNSELOR	"I notice that people look to me when they talk." ■ GIVING FEEDBACK ● to acknowledge ▼ group behavior
2	COUNSELOR	"I see heads nodding." ■ GIVING FEEDBACK ● to acknowledge ▼ group behavior
3	COUNSELOR	"I hear this side of the room saying they want to stop." ■ GIVING FEEDBACK ● to acknowledge ▼ subgroup behavior

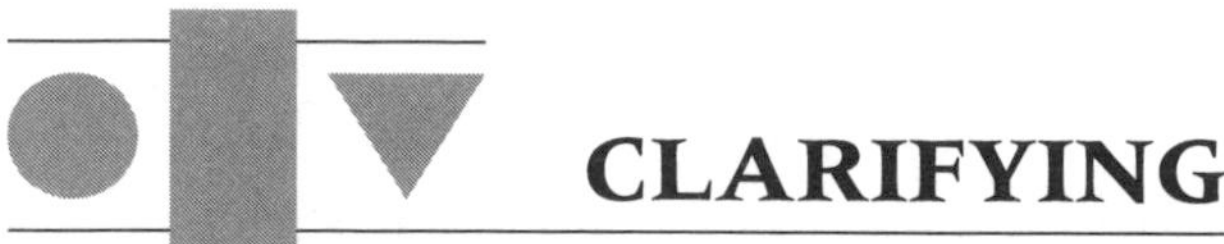

CLARIFYING

TYPE OF RESPONSE
ACTIVE

CLARIFYING is a response from the counselor to encourage the client(s) to be clear about what he/she is truly feeling and experiencing. As a result, the client(s) becomes more aware, and less vague. A client(s) will use generalizations and abstract notions to avoid the focus and defend against anxiety. As the counselor asks the client(s) to clarify and be more concrete, these defenses are confronted. It is *not* the counselor's job to do the clarifying for the client(s).

If the counselor is unclear about what the client(s) is saying, the client(s) may also be unclear. The counselor should not make assumptions. Therefore, asking for clarification can be for both the client(s) and the counselor. A client(s) may say, "I'm depressed." The counselor should not assume that either the client or the counselor understands what this means and ask for clarification, for example, "What do you mean by 'depressed'?"

Initially, CLARIFYING should be used with caution to avoid interrupting and distracting. Later, especially in planning and action phases of counseling, it may be necessary to clarify often and to encourage exactness.

Though it may be a challenge for the client(s) to clarify responses, the intent of the counselor is almost always to encourage exploration of a vague or incomplete statement by the client(s). The focus of CLARIFYING is on experience, feeling, thought, or behavior. However, in CLARIFYING responses, the words of the counselor may not indicate focus since they often only refer to what the client(s) is saying. Often the client(s) is talking about an experience, and to encourage clarification of the broader experience, the counselor will respond with a narrower focus on feelings, thoughts or behaviors.

Asking the client(s) to clarify can also be done by requesting that the client(s) tell you *more* about what he/she is talking about. You are not asking specifically for more concrete or specific information. Such CLARIFYING responses may be in the form of a question, "Will you tell me *more* about that?" or a statement of short words such as "uh-huh," or nods of the head, or short sentences or phrases such as, "Tell me more about that." This may sound like DIRECTING, that is, telling the client(s) what to do, but it does not ask for a change of direction for something new, just something more. The response may also be words followed by an ellipsis such as "and . . . " or "and then . . . " This type of CLARIFYING response encourages the client(s) to disclose personal information and indicates a willingness on the part of the counselor to listen. The intent of this type of CLARIFYING is to encourage the client(s) to tell *more;* that is, to expand on what he/she is saying.

CLARIFYING in Groups

Especially in a group, CLARIFYING encourages interaction among members as they expand on their thoughts and feelings. The secondary value is other members of the group (and the counselor) will have a clearer picture of what is being communicated. As an active response, group members are expected to react to the counselor's request for clarification. In doing so, group members learn more about each other in a more concrete way, thus promoting group interaction and cohesiveness. Increased clarification can also escalate the knowledge of similarities and differences among members. Jacobs, Masson, Harvill (1998) state the following:

> Often, the leader will find it necessary to help members clarify their statements. Clarification may be done for the benefit of the entire group or for the speaker's benefit—that is, to help the member become more aware of what he or she is trying to say (p. 115).

EXAMPLES OF CLARIFYING IN GROUPS

1	COUNSELOR	"Talk more about what it feels like to terminate." ■ CLARIFYING ● to explore ▼ group feeling
2.1	CLIENT A	"I don't know! You are the counselor; you should have it all put together."
2.2	CLIENT B	"You know, you should know what to talk about."
2.3	COUNSELOR	"Can you tell me more about 'I should know'?" ■ CLARIFYING ● to explore ▼ individual feeling *Note that it is in question form, though it is really asking for expansion rather than new information.*

DIRECTING

TYPE OF RESPONSE
ACTIVE

As the counseling relationship becomes more trusting and rapport has been established, it may be appropriate for the counselor to be directive. To be directive is to ask the client to do something new or different or to go in a different direction. The counselor may ask the client(s) to go back to something that was said earlier, or to stop and stay with an emotion. Giving homework is another way of DIRECTING. When asking the client(s) to respond to a specific direction, the counselor should be mindful of the client(s)' reaction to the directive. The counselor should be respectful of the client(s)' willingness and readiness to engage in the activity.

To be directive is not to ask for more information, though it may often sound like a directive; for example, "Tell me more" (CLARIFYING). QUESTIONING or CLARIFYING responses with the intent to explore, and asked after the carrying out of a directive, can help the client(s) understand and internalize the impact of the question. For example, the counselor can say, "How was it for you to do this exercise?" or "Tell me how it is when I ask you to stay with this?"

DIRECTING is usually done with the intent to explore or to challenge. By asking the client(s) to engage in a new activity, the counselor may intend for the client(s) to explore an area of interest or further explore their current situation, behavior or feeling. The result of the direction can be quite challenging for the client(s); that may also be the intent of the counselor's directive. Asking the client(s) to dialogue with an empty chair will most often challenge the client(s) to consider different thoughts or beliefs, feelings, or behaviors.

DIRECTING in Groups

DIRECTING is extremely important in group counseling. The group counselor, by DIRECTING, can influence the course of the group and the extent of the interaction among clients. Because DIRECTING is, literally, telling the group or members of the group what to do, the counselor's "power" to "direct" the group dynamics is most felt using this response.

The counselor can direct the group as a whole. This may be done to set up or reinforce certain norms or to involve the group in certain activities or exercises. DIRECTING a group of people rather than an individual can result in increased resistance and, on the contrary, increased involvement. Group counselors must be aware of the impact that a directive can have on the group.

One valuable use of DIRECTING is to facilitate the significant variable of clients hearing from and responding to each other. As noted in other descriptions of counseling responses, the counselor can direct clients to give almost any counseling response to each other or to the group as a whole. The counselor can, by DIRECTING, have one member GIVING FEEDBACK to another; PARAPHRASING what the group is experiencing; or QUESTIONING the group. Again, since group members have so much influence on each other, DIRECTING the interaction among group members is an important counselor task. DIRECTING is not questioning, but may be stated in the form of a question or request: Could this side of the group tell the other side how they are reacting right now?"

Example 3 below exemplifies Yalom's (1995) concept of the "self-reflective loop":

> . . . The effective use of the here-and-now requires two steps; the group lives in the here and now and it also doubles back on itself: it performs a self-reflective loop and examines the here-and-now behavior that has just occurred (p. 130).

There are many terms that describe directive responses. They refer to an active intervention or confrontation by the counselor. *Blocking* is an example of a directive group counseling response as defined in Corey (2000):

> Blocking refers to the leader's intervention to stop counterproductive behaviors within the group. It is a skill that requires sensitivity, directness, and the ability to stop the activity without attacking the person (p. 44).

EXAMPLES OF DIRECTING IN GROUPS

1	COUNSELOR	"I'd like to stop the group here and go back to this question of some members not feeling heard." ■ DIRECTING ● to challenge ▼ subgroup behavior
2	COUNSELOR	"I would like the group to use 'I' statements instead of 'you.'" ■ DIRECTING ● to challenge ▼ group behavior
3	COUNSELOR	"I want to stop the group here and ask you how it felt to share this with each other right here in the group." ■ DIRECTING ● to challenge ▼ group behavior and ■ QUESTIONING ● to challenge ▼ group feeling with immediacy in context *Note the use of both DIRECTING and QUESTIONING to get the group to focus on what just happened in the group, adding both immediacy and context.*

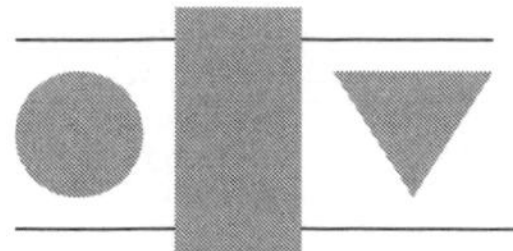

QUESTIONING

TYPE OF RESPONSE
ACTIVE

QUESTIONING can challenge the client(s) to evaluate whether behaviors, thoughts, or feelings are effective in getting what he/she wants; for example, "How is this working for you?" "How" questions often evoke responses in which the client(s) has to reflect upon new or existing information. When the client(s) presents feeling different one week from the next, a counselor could ask, "How is this week different from last week?"

Asking questions to get information is a response that most people have mastered. The counselor, however, should have a therapeutic intent, that is, to acknowledge, to explore, or to challenge the client(s), rather than just to get information. Most QUESTIONING as a counseling response is done with the intent to challenge. "How" questions are usually open ended—"How do you feel about that?" "Why" questions are also open ended, but require an appropriate rationale and can put the client(s) on the defense. Counselors are encouraged not to ask double questions, "Is it hard for you to both work and study, and how does your family feel about this?" Note that this question is not only double, but the focus is on both the client(s) and other people; it also asks for a feeling response and for information. Counselors are also encouraged not to ask a question and then give a multiple-choice answer as this inhibits client(s) exploration; for example, "How do you feel about that; sad, confused, angry . . .?"

Refraining from asking questions is not easy. The counselor needs to know the importance of timing: when to ask a question and when not to ask a question. Timing is learned by having some understanding of the therapeutic value of the question and the anticipated response from the client(s).

The client(s) often does not respond to the counselor's question. The counselor, if he/she wants the client(s) to respond to the question, may need to follow up by repeating the question or GIVING FEEDBACK—"I notice that you did not respond to my question."

While QUESTIONING is named as a distinct basic counseling response, other basic counseling responses can be in the form of a question; for example, "How would you like to start the session?" (OPENING or CLOSING) or "can you be more specific or give an example?" (CLARIFYING).

Questions can be either open-ended or close-ended. An open-ended question generally elicits two or three sentences; a close-ended question can usually be answered with one or two words. As a counseling response, open-ended questions usually evoke more exploration. The focus can be on feeling, experience, thoughts or behavior, as well as immediacy.

QUESTIONING in Groups

QUESTIONING is a very important response in group counseling. Questions are the most often used response in group counseling. Corey (2000) notes that QUESTIONING can be overused:

> Questioning is probably the technique that the novice group leaders tend to overuse the most. Bombarding members with question after question does not lead to productive outcomes and may even have a negative affect on the group interaction (p. 39).

While this is true, very often the group counselor is QUESTIONING to challenge the group members themselves to use the other responses. For example, if a counselor prefers members GIVING FEEDBACK to an individual, subgroup, or group, instead of the counselor giving the response, the counselor will elicit the feedback from the group by asking a question such as, "How is the group reacting to the way Brenda is speaking right now?" The "power of group" is that there are peers in the group who can give a variety of responses that often have much more impact than if the counselor made the response.

Using questions in tandem, with different focuses, is what the authors of this text have been calling the *one-two punch.* The one-two punch is a way to focus on an individual in the context of the group, and then question the group so that they can respond to their experience and to the issue presented by the individual. This combination of responses can only be done in a group.

EXAMPLES OF QUESTIONING IN GROUPS

1	COUNSELOR	"What does the group want to do with this issue of confidentiality?" ■ QUESTIONING ● to challenge ▼ group behavior
2	COUNSELOR	"How does the group feel about Susan wanting to drop out of the group?" ■ QUESTIONING ● to challenge ▼ group feeling
3.1	COUNSELOR	"When you think about ending this group when you don't want to, and you're not ready, how does that compare to other situations where you've had to say goodbye?" ■ QUESTIONING ● to challenge ▼ group thought *This question is designed to relate the group experience to other experiences. Yalom (1995) uses the terms family reenactmen and group as a social microcosm to describe the phenomena such a question may measure. This is an especially powerful question when a group is terminating.*
3.2	CLIENT A	"School, when you leave for the summer."
3.3	CLIENT B	"Well, when my dad died. 'Cause I thought he'd be there when I was older, a lot older."
4	COUNSELOR	"What does it mean to other members of the group when Sally said that she is hurt by what was said?" ■ QUESTIONING ● to challenge ▼ group thought *This is an example of asking for meaning in a question form. It could be argued that this is CLARIFYING to explore group feeling or it could be that the counselor is DIRECTING the group for GIVING FEEDBACK to Sally.*

EXAMPLES OF THE ONE-TWO PUNCH IN GROUPS

5	COUNSELOR	"How did it feel for you to share this with the group?" *Allow time for the client to respond, then add,* "How was it for the group to hear her say this?" ■ QUESTIONING ● to challenge ▼ individual feeling in context ■ QUESTIONING ● to challenge ▼ group feeling *Note: The "in context" in the first question is because the counselor used the words "with the group," which substantially changes the question. The question to the group assumes the context of the group.*

6.1	COUNSELOR	"Debbie, I'm wondering how it has been for you to have a lot of focus and a lot of energy directed towards you and the issues you brought up?" ■ QUESTIONING ● to challenge ▼ individual experience
6.2	CLIENT A (Debbie)	"That's a good question because while I was driving over here, I was thinking about how last week the focus towards the end of the meeting has been kind of on me. And how much I hate focus being on me for any reason. And so, uh, although I have had great insight here, it has been really hard for me to have . . . to have you be aware of me. I am more comfortable if I'm just sitting here and not having people aware of and thinking about me."
6.3	CLIENT B	"But this whole being here is about growth. And growth hurts. Growth stinks (laughs). Don't ya think?" (to Debbie)
6.4	CLIENT C	"Well, it's focus of any type, even compliments. I feel very uncomfort able when people pay me compliments. So, it's focus of any kind. So, it's uncomfortable, to say the least."
6.5	COUNSELOR	"I wonder how it's been for the group to focus a lot of energy on Debbie and what's been going on for her?" ■ QUESTIONING ● to challenge ▼ group experience

7.1	CLIENT	"Gosh, I'm glad this is coming to an end. You know, its kind of revisiting those hard feelings again."
7.2	COUNSELOR	"How are you feeling in your body right now?" ■ QUESTIONING ● to challenge ▼ individual feeling with immediacy
7.3	CLIENT	"Um, relieved . . . kind of lighter . . . kind of drained. More drained than anything."
7.4	COUNSELOR	"How is the rest of the group feeling right now?" ■ QUESTIONING ● to challenge ▼ group feeling with immediacy *Note how the counselor focused on the individual client and then brought the focus back to the group.*

PLAYING A HUNCH, REFRAMING

TYPE OF RESPONSE
INTERPRETIVE

PLAYING A HUNCH requires that a level of trust has been established between the client(s) and the counselor, and that the counselor trusts his/her intuitive sense of "what *might* be going on." PLAYING A HUNCH is used to lead to a deeper understanding of client(s) issues, feelings, or situation, and the meaning that the client(s) gives to them. Thus, over a period of time, the counselor forms an interpretation, shares this with the client(s), encourages the processing of this new information and, when appropriate, asks the client(s) to reflect on the experience of processing the new information. A hunch does not have to be accurate; a hunch is what the counselor feels, and might not be what the client(s) feels. The importance of a hunch is to give the client(s) an opportunity to react to some new information.

The intent is to challenge the client(s). The focus can be on experience, feeling, client(s) thought and/or behavior, and have an immediacy focus. Hunches can be played with tentativeness because they are interpretations and often confrontational.

REFRAMING gives the client(s) another view on experience, feelings, thought, behavior, or the current situation. Often, the client(s) can see the variables of their lives only from their own perspective; the more objective counselor often can see things differently. The counselor, using data from the client(s), offers an alternative explanation or interpretation of areas of focus:

- An experience: "I wonder if this can be seen as an opportunity to make a change"; or
- A feeling: "You say 'anxiety,' but another word may be 'excitement'";
- A thought: "You say that you haven't learned anything from this experience, but you have learned how to survive"; and/or
- A behavior: "This feeling may be a signal to avoid the situation."

The counselor may have a very different focus than that of the client(s) since the idea is to offer an alternative view of the issue. REFRAMING is an invitation to look at something differently. Because it comes from the counselor and is both interpretive and confrontational, it can be offered tentatively. REFRAMING is intended to challenge the client(s) to consider a different perspective. The focus can be on his/her feeling, experience, or behavior, and be an immediacy focus.

REFRAMING and PLAYING A HUNCH are often very close in intent and delivery. Both are designed to present new information and both depend on the counselor to go beyond what the client(s) is saying. REFRAMING is to suggest an alternative viewpoint; PLAYING A HUNCH is to share the counselor's own interpretation of what may be the case.

PLAYING A HUNCH in Groups

PLAYING A HUNCH is probably the most interpretive response that counselors make. The hunch is the counselor's guess of what "might be." This is difficult with an individual client, and even more speculative with a group. In a group, hunches may provoke discussion, disagreement, and a challenge to the counselor. The sharing of hunches in a group can give new information or possible explanations for members' experience. Group members may then build upon the counselor's hunch. For example, the counselor may say, "I have a hunch that it might be scary to talk about the anger that people feel in the group." Members may offer other hunches, such as "It might be that we just don't know where to start" or "I think we might be afraid to hurt other people's feelings."

In his discussion of "mass group commentary," and specifically a group tendency toward "flight" from painful issues, Yalom (1995) says:

> The precise nature and timing of the intervention is largely a matter of individual style. Some therapists, myself included tend to intervene when they sense a presence of group flight even though they do not clearly understand its source. I may for example, comment that I feel puzzled or uneasy about the meeting and inquire, "Is there something the group is not talking about today?" or "Is the group avoiding something?" or "I have a sense there's a 'hidden agenda' today; could we talk about this?" (p. 180).

The therapist's "sense of a presence" is the hunch—the forming of a hunch germinates from the feelings of puzzlement or uneasiness. PLAYING A HUNCH is the statement "I have a sense there's a 'hidden agenda' today . . ." (Note: The other hunches are QUESTIONING and have a different impact as the clients must answer the question versus other possible reactions that a non-question hunch may generate.)

EXAMPLES OF PLAYING A HUNCH IN GROUPS

1	COUNSELOR	"I have a hunch that the group really wants to deal with this, but is afraid of hurting each others' feelings." ■ PLAYING A HUNCH ● to challenge ▼ group feelings

2	COUNSELOR	"It seems like some of you talk about other people outside the room so you don't have to get too close to each other." ■ PLAYING A HUNCH ● to challenge ▼ subgroup behavior

3.1	CLIENT A	"I don't think Marcy (Client 2) is being passive because she has been offering us a lot of advise, being very active in the group and asking us a lot of questions."
3.2	CLIENT B	"She's helping everyone else in the group but not revealing her true self."
3.3	COUNSELOR	"I have a hunch that some group members try to help so that the focus doesn't have to be on them and they don't have to reveal their true selves." ■ PLAYING A HUNCH ● to challenge ▼ subgroup behavior

4.1	CLIENT A	"Maybe we can make a note that we all meet at the diner down the road. Does that sound like a good idea?"
4.2	CLIENT B	"Everybody pitch in for drinks and stuff and talk about their problems."
4.3	CLIENT C	"Oh, yeah. You know what I think, they should have. Since we won't be meeting . . . I think they should have a camp or something."
4.4	COUNSELOR	"It sounds like you guys are not quite ready to have the group end." ■ PLAYING A HUNCH ● to challenge ▼ group experience

REFRAMING in Groups

The group counselor must be aware of what the group is saying and be able to offer an alternative view. Because other group members tend to do this easily with each other, the group counselor does not often reframe for individuals in a group. There are, however, times when the counselor is aware that the group as a whole could consider an alternative view of what is being said or experienced in the group. It is the counselor's view that is being offered as an alternative to the group expression, thus making this response both interpretive and, possibly, at odds with the group's position. Any reframe, however, increases the range of the group's understanding of its own dynamic.

EXAMPLES OF REFRAMING IN GROUPS

1	COUNSELOR	"Another way of looking at this conflict is that there is an opportunity to resolve this among yourselves." ■ REFRAMING ● to challenge ▼ group behavior
2	COUNSELOR	". . . or, with the differences among you, you can better understand your own issues from a different perspective." ■ REFRAMING ● to challenge ▼ group thought

NOTING A THEME, NOTING A CONNECTION, NOTING A DISCREPANCY

TYPE OF RESPONSE
INTERPRETIVE

A counselor often looks for themes or patterns that run through the session or a series of sessions: themes of interacting, behaving, thinking, and feeling. For example, the counselor might point out that whenever the client(s) gets into difficult situations he/she tries to escape, run away, or leave the situation. This would be a pattern noticed over a period of time. NOTING A THEME needs to be clearly stated and thus can be confrontational. As with other responses that require that the counselor be more interpretive, tentative language can be used. The intent of NOTING A THEME could be to acknowledge or to explore, but more often it is to challenge the client(s). Counselors may choose to use the word *theme* or *pattern*, rather than just responding to what has been heard, which may be closer to the response of PARAPHRASING. NOTING A THEME is not just pointing out a common denominator or a repeated topic, but impressing on the client(s) the significance of frequent occurrence of a theme that they may not be aware of. The client(s) often does not see apparent discrepancies or apparent connections; the counselor, being more objective, can.

NOTING A DISCREPANCY and NOTING A CONNECTION are similar. They both can be confrontational; each requires the counselor to compare different things that the client(s) has said and to present these to the client(s). The difference is that discrepancies don't seem to go together; connections do.

Connections can include *similarities* between:

- What a client(s) is saying *or not saying* and the counselor's perception of what the client(s) is experiencing;
- What the client(s) is saying and what the counselor heard the client(s) say at any time; or
- What the client(s) is saying in the session and the client(s)' actions outside the session.

As in NOTING A DISCREPANCY, the intent is to challenge; the focus can be on feeling, experience, and/or behavior and immediacy. Using NOTING A DISCREPANCY or NOTING A THEME, the counselor can choose to be more explicit: " I see a connection . . . "; or more tentative: "It seems that there may be a connection between . . . "

Discrepancies or apparent discrepancies are pointed out by the counselor from what the counselor has observed and surmised. In other words, the counselor goes beyond what the client(s) has recently said, and suggests that there may be a discrepancy in what the client(s) is now saying, has said before, or is doing. For example, "I notice that a few minutes ago you said that you wanted to change; now you are saying that you do not want to change." Note that "but" was not used, which makes this confrontation "softer." A "harder" confrontation may be used when a softer confrontation has not been recognized. For example, "You said that you wanted to change, but now you are saying . . . "; note that *but* was used. In both of the previous examples the discrepancy is implied. Though the response may actually sound like GIVING FEEDBACK or PARAPHRASING, the counselor's intent—to challenge rather than to acknowledge—is what defines the NOTING A DISCREPANCY response. Stronger use of this response might entail the actual use of the word discrepancy; for example, "I see a discrepancy between . . . " A slightly softer response may use tentativeness: "It seems that there may be a discrepancy between . . . "

Confrontation is almost always an integral part of the interpretive responses, especially NOTING A DISCREPANCY. Thus, any of the interpretive responses could be confrontational in that the counselor presents new information or known information in a new way.

NOTING A DISCREPANCY means that the counselor must trust his/her own awareness and the ability of the client(s) to process the apparent discrepancy. It is helpful to follow up a discrepancy with an opportunity for the client(s) to discuss the impact of having a discrepancy noted, "How was it to have this pointed out?" (QUESTIONING with the intent to challenge.)

Discrepancies can include *differences* between:

- What a client(s) is saying *or not saying* and the counselor's perception of what the client(s) is experiencing;
- What the client(s) is saying and what the counselor heard the client(s) say at another time;
- What the client(s) is saying in the session and the client(s)' actions outside the session; or
- What the client(s) is saying that is not congruent with the client(s)' behavior.

Because a discrepancy usually involves two components, counselors often use both hands ("On one hand . . . on the other . . . ") to express these two components. This nonverbal expression assists in the presentation of both what appears to be a discrepancy as well as components that seem to be connected.

The intent of NOTING A DISCREPANCY is almost always to challenge. The counselor is not pointing out two or more issues that may or may not be congruent (this would be GIVING FEEDBACK), but rather that there appears, to the counselor, to be a discrepancy. The focus of this response can be the feeling, thought, and/or behavior and can be, additionally, the focus of immediacy. This type of response may have multiple focuses because the counselor is pointing out discrepant components.

NOTING A THEME, NOTING A CONNECTION, and NOTING A DISCREPENCY in Groups

In groups, the opportunity for NOTING A THEME, NOTING A CONNECTION, and NOTING A DISCREPENCY abound. Group counselors can help members of the group become aware of themes running through a group, connections among members, and discrepancies within the group. Noting these can help an individual to better understand who they are in relationship to other group members. As the group as a whole becomes more aware of both similarities and differences, several things can happen: The group becomes cohesive because of connections and often accepts differences and discrepancies.

Because of the number of people in a group, there may be a variety of themes. As cohesion grows, common themes emerge. Likewise, as the counselor notes common themes, members become aware of their similarities, their universality and cohesion can occur. Of universality, Yalom (1995) says:

> After hearing other members disclose concerns similar to their own, patients report feeling more in touch with the world and describe the process as a "welcome to the human race" experience. Simply put, this phenomena finds expression in the cliché 'We're all in the same boat . . .' (p. 6).

Corey (2000) speaks to the overlap of NOTING A THEME and NOTING A CONNECTION:

> One way of promoting interaction among members is to look for themes that emerge in the group and then to connect the work that members do with these themes. Through linking several members together, the leader also teaches them how to take responsibility for involving themselves in the work of others (p. 44).

As group members start to self-disclose, the counselor can see connections between how members are feeling and commonalities in their experiences. The same is true of discrepancies. The more members know of each other, the more differences will become evident, and the more opportunity the counselor has to note these. Differences may result in conflict, a predictable phenomena in groups. Discrepancies in a group may be expressed in contrary feelings, values, and opinions. As with themes and connections, as members learn of differences between themselves and others, they can learn to better understand their position in the group and in their own out-of-group lives. Yalom (1995) speaks to this dynamic:

> As members are able to go beyond the mere statement of position as they begin to understand the other's experiential world, past and present, and view the other's position from their own frame of reference, they begin to understand that the other's point of view may be as appropriate for that person as their own is for themselves (p. 65).

These three counseling responses all require that the counselor actually name the theme, the connections, or the discrepancies. The counselor is in a position to see and sense these dynamics because the counselor is apart from the group, observing the group, and attending to the many varied verbal and nonverbal expressions not necessarily seen or heard by the clients. They will, however, begin to model these responses, especially in the later stages of a group.

Because of the interpretive nature of these responses, they may overlap. The counselor may have a hunch that there is a connection or see a connection between themes, as shown in the examples below. When this happens, the first response may be the most identifiable:

"I have this sense that there is a connection between this issue of self-disclosure and the comfort level in the group."

PLAYING A HUNCH to challenge feeling in context

"There seems to be a relationship between the theme of 'when will this end' and 'we're ready to get on with our lives.'"

NOTING A CONNECTION to challenge group feeling

EXAMPLES OF NOTING A THEME IN GROUPS

1	COUNSELOR	"There is a theme of 'we are all in this together' right now, in this group." ■ NOTING A THEME ● to challenge ▼ group feeling *In context with immediacy in context*
2	COUNSELOR	"There is a theme of 'we will not challenge each other' in the group." ■ NOTING A THEME ● to challenge ▼ group feeling in context
3.1	CLIENT A	"Um, yes . . . I've tried to talk to them. He knows what we feel and he knows why. But he doesn't think there's anything wrong. He can do what he wants to do because he works, he pays the bills."
3.2	CLIENT B	"Right. But I have to limit my daughter's phone calls. And I've told her that. I told her, 'You do make me anxious and I'm in this mess because I can't handle your problems.'"
3.3	COUNSELOR	"I keep hearing a theme from many of you saying, 'I have no control.'" ■ NOTING A THEME ● to challenge ▼ subgroup behavior

EXAMPLES OF NOTING A CONNECTION IN GROUPS

1	COUNSELOR	"I see a connection between how willing people are to share and the level of trust among you." ■ NOTING A CONNECTION ● to challenge ▼ group behavior and feelings
2	COUNSELOR	"I notice a relationship between the topic we are talking about and a hesitancy to respond." ■ NOTING A CONNECTION ● to challenge ▼ group behavior

EXAMPLES OF NOTING A DISCREPANCY IN GROUPS

1	COUNSELOR	"There seems to be a discrepancy between what the group says they want to talk about and your willingness to self disclose." ■ NOTING A DISCREPANCY ● to challenge ▼ group behavior
2	COUNSELOR	"Last week the group said that they thought that everything said here is confidential, yet this issue was brought up during the break." ■ NOTING A DISCREPANCY ● to challenge ▼ group thought and behavior *Note the double focus.*
3.1	CLIENT A	"Yeah. I'm trying to act like an adult."
3.2	CLIENT B	"This is a group for teens."
3.3	CLIENT A	"I know, but I like to act like an adult. It makes me feel more like one."
3.4	CLIENT C	"I just say whatever I want."
3.5	COUNSELOR	"I hear people saying that they feel comfortable, but I am also feeling a little tension in the room. Some group members are doing a lot more talking, while others are pretty quiet." ■ NOTING A DISCREPANCY ● to challenge ▼ group and subgroup feeling and behavior *Note the double focus.*
3.6	CLIENT A	"Well, I know I can't say whatever I want. It wouldn't be right."

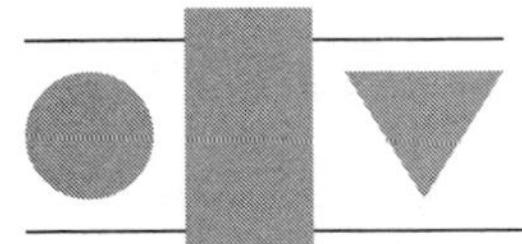

ALLOWING SILENCE

TYPE OF RESPONSE
DISCRETIONARY

Silence is the art of knowing when to be quiet. It is knowing, from ATTENDING, when it is more important to let the client(s) process internally rather than verbally. It is believing that it is not the counselor's responsibility to either be talking or to keep the client(s) talking. It is also knowing when to break the silence (and when to allow the client(s) to break the silence) and when to ask the client(s), for example, "What was going on during that silence?" Silence is verbal silence, which means that nodding, for example, may be appropriate. On the other hand, it may also mean not keeping eye contact to give "space."

The counselor needs to think about the timing of being silent as an intentional response—it is not always appropriate. Some client(s) comments need immediate acknowledgment from the counselor. Silence is most useful when the client(s) is engaged in self-analysis, which can be helpful to achieve one goal of counseling—client(s) self-awareness.

The intent of ALLOWING SILENCE generally is to allow the client(s) to explore, within themselves, the issue being discussed. The counselor could also intentionally allow silence to challenge the client(s) to come up with a response that could grow out of the silence. The focus of silence is always on the client(s), but is not easily differentiated between client(s) feelings, client(s) thought, and client(s) behavior.

ALLOWING SILENCE in Groups

There is less silence in a group than individual counseling because there are more people in the group to break the silence. Referring to breaking the silence, Carrol and Wiggins (1997) say,

> One of the major fears of group leaders is to encounter silence from members. If this happens, what does the leader do? What does the leader say? Does the leader just let the silence go on and on, and thereby put pressure on the group? (p. 49).

The counseling response of ALLOWING SILENCE is made when the counselor chooses not to break the silence, but rather, to deliberately not make a verbal response because the counselor feels the group needs the time to contemplate or reflect, or that the group needs to take the responsibility to break the silence.

EXAMPLE OF ALLOWING SILENCE IN GROUPS

1	COUNSELOR	(The group is waiting for someone to comment and the counselor chooses not to be the one.) ■ ALLOWING SILENCE ● to acknowledge ▼ group behavior

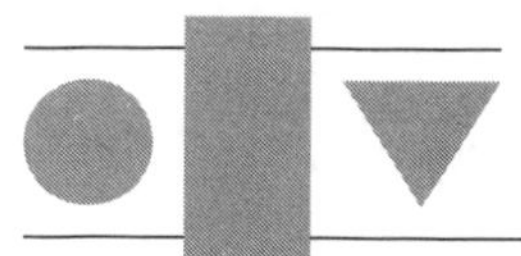

SELF-DISCLOSING

TYPE OF RESPONSE
DISCRETIONARY

SELF-DISCLOSING is probably the most difficult response to understand because it requires that the counselor know when and how much information about the counselor might benefit the client(s). Also, the counselor must be able to keep the focus on the client(s) even though the counselor is sharing personal information. The counselor must be aware of transference and countertransference dynamics and the effect, therapeutically, of self-disclosure on those dynamics.

The intent of SELF-DISCLOSING is to acknowledge; the focus is on the counselor, though only temporarily. Should the client(s) want to know more about the counselor's disclosure, the counselor may choose to respond with, "How is it for you to hear my experience?" (QUESTIONING with the intent to challenge that puts the focus back on the client(s).)

SELF-DISCLOSING in Groups

The group counselor can use his/her own reactions and feelings about the group to help the group examine their own feelings and give permission to speak about uncomfortable things. Yalom (1995) makes two significant and related points regarding self-disclosure in groups:

> Self-disclosure is absolutely mandatory in the group therapeutic process (p. 120).
>
> Therapist self-disclosure is an aid to the group members because it sets a model for the patients and permits some patients to reality-test their feelings toward you (p. 216).

Thus, the group counselor would choose SELF-DISCLOSING because it is necessary for members to self-disclose and the counselor models this behavior. Therefore, the counselor should self-disclose for the benefit of the group. The counselor does not self-disclose for the counselor's benefit; the counselor is not a member of the group and the counselor's role is not to participate as a member.

In addition to modeling as Yalom (1995) suggests, SELF-DISCLOSING can be either a confirmation of the group experience or an alternative to the group experience:

I was nervous in my first group experience."
SELF-DISCLOSING to acknowledge group feelings
This may validate the feelings of group members.

If someone said that to me I would be angry.
SELF-DISCLOSING to challenge group feelings
The counselor suggests a possible alternative.

EXAMPLES OF SELF-DISCLOSING IN GROUPS

1	COUNSELOR	"When I'm in a new group situation I often have the fear of other people judging me." ■ SELF-DISCLOSING ● to challenge ▼ group feelings
2	COUNSELOR	"I feel uncomfortable with the group giving advice." ■ SELF-DISCLOSING ● to challenge ▼ group behavior

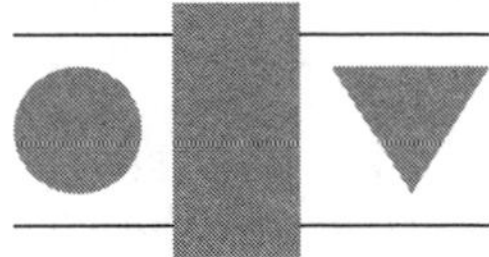

PART 3
Exercises

This section includes:

- Introduction
- The Groups
- Using the CD-ROM
- Accessing the Web site
- Exercises for the videocassette
- Advanced exercises

Introduction

The exercises are designed to help students identify, create, and demonstrate counseling RESPONSES, intents, and focuses in groups.

- Videocassette Exercises 1 and 2 are to be used with the worktext and videocassette.
- CD-ROM Exercises 1–5 are on the CD-ROM.
- Advanced Exercises 1–5 are in this section of the worktext.
- Video examples of counseling responses are available on the CD-ROM.
- The number of the group corresponds with the number of the exercise on both the videocassette and the CD-ROM. For example, Group 1/women is both on the Videocassette Exercise 1 and CD-ROM Exercise 1. The exercises, however, are not the same.

Complete transcripts of Group 1/women and Group 2/boys are with the respective videocassette exercises. Transcripts of Group 3/graduates, Group 4/students, and Group 5/adults (CD-ROM only) are in Appendix A. Suggested identifications of counseling RESPONSES, intents, and focuses are included in the transcripts except for the selections used for the exercises. For these selections, the identifications follow the transcripts so that students can compare their own identifications with the suggested ones. Table 5 shows how the groups and exercises are distributed between the videocassette, the worktext, and the CD-ROM.

TABLE 5: WORKTEXT/VIDEOCASSETTE AND CD-ROM EXERCISES

EXERCISE	NUMBER OF IDENTIFICATIONS/ SELECTIONS	VIDEOCASSETTE AND WORKTEXT	CD-ROM	TRANSCRIPTS
Worktext/ videocassette				
1	16	Group 1/women, sessions a, b, c		Worktext, p. 64
2	12	Group 2/boys		Worktext, p. 84
CD-ROM				
1	8		Clips: Group 1/women, sessions a and b	Worktext, pp. 68, 70, 76–77
2	13		Clips: Group 2/boys	Worktext, pp. 88–89, 91, 99–100, 110–112
3	8		Group 3/graduates	Appendix A
4	10		Group 4/students	Appendix A
5	11		Group 5/adults	Appendix A
Worktext Advanced 1–5				

The sessions are not meant to be ideal. In all exercises, critique is encouraged. The suggested identifications of RESPONSES, intents, and focuses, as well as the comments, should be seen as open for discussion and debate.

On both the videocassette and CD-ROM, each group session or clip opens with an identification of the group in the center of the screen. The counselor and clients will be identified on the screen at this time. In groups with multiple sessions, each session will be identified separately. When the counselor is speaking, the number of the counselor response appears on the left. When a group member is speaking, the number of the member response appears on the right. When a group is co-counseled, counselors are identified as counselor A and counselor B in the opening of the session, in the group diagram, and in the transcripts, but only the number of the response appears on the screen. Group members are identified by name as the session opens, in the group diagram, and in the transcript. As with the counselors, only the number appears on the screen. The diagrams for each group are in Appendix A.

The videocassette and CD-ROM exercises require that the student:

- OBSERVE the interaction (all exercises)
- IDENTIFY RESPONSE, intent, and focus (all exercises except CD-ROM Exercises 1 and 2)
- CREATE responses (CD-ROM Exercises 1–5)

- COMPARE selected identifications with the suggested identifications (all exercises except CD-ROM Exercises 1 and 2); COMPARE a changed response with other possibilities (CD-ROM Exercises 1 and 2) or COMPARE created responses with the actual responses (CD-ROM Exercises 3, 4, and 5);
- DEMONSTRATE counseling responses (Advanced Exercises 1–5)
- REFLECT: Reflection questions that refer to the content and process of the group sessions, group counseling ethics, group development, and diversity in groups (Videocassette Exercises 1 and 2 and Advanced Exercises 1–5).
- NOTE BOX: Each CD-ROM exercise has a box in which the student can make process comments or ask questions. The process comments and questions can be saved and for example, be included in a portfolio, printed, or e-mailed to the instructor or other students.

The Groups

- All group sessions were unscripted and unrehearsed.
- The tapes were edited for length.
- None of the groups met before.
- Clients were all volunteers.
- Some clients had prior group counseling experience.
- Clients are identified by name, although many clients chose to use an alias.
- Clients and counselors represent a variety of ethnic and cultural backgrounds.

All groups were given a short orientation to the group experience. Adult clients chose the type of group that they wanted to be part of and wrote their personal goals for their group experience prior to the sessions. Examples of goal statements can be found in Appendix A of this worktext.

All groups started with introductions, the sharing of goals, and an explanation of confidentiality. These portions of the groups were edited out for time, but an example of the confidentiality discussion from Group 5/adults can be found in Appendix A. Also refer to *The Making of the Basic Counseling Responses in Groups Video,* preface, page x.

- Group 1/women (sessions a, b, and c) is a women's group similar to those offered by community agencies. This group met three times. The three sessions show how a group moves through stages of group development. The seven clients represent a variety of backgrounds; some cultural differences are discussed in the sessions. Major themes of this group are guilt, selfishness, and anger. The three sessions of this group are all presented in the Videocassette Exercise 1. Selected clips are on the CD-ROM Exercise 1.
- Group 2/boys is a group of 13- to 17-year-old males from an adolescent treatment program. The group demonstrates movement from "chaos" to "cohesion" within one session. A major shift from the dominant members of the group to the less dominant members is evident. This session in its entirety is in Videocassette Exercise 2 and clips are on CD-ROM Exercise 2.
- Group 3/graduates is a group of male and female graduate students in a group similar to one that might be offered by a university counseling center. This session is co-counseled. The stress of being a graduate student and conflict with the counselors are discussed in this session. This group is presented in CD-ROM Exercise 3.
- Group 4/students is an anger management, psycho-educational group like those that might be offered in a middle or junior high school. The group counselor demonstrates how counseling

responses can be used in a structured group format. There are two male and four female students in this group. This group is presented in CD-ROM Exercise 4.

- Group 5/adults is a first session of a group that could be offered by a community agency for individuals wanting to work on relationships in a group counseling situation. The group is co-counseled and co-educational. This group depicts both conflict and conflict resolution. The complete group session is in CD-ROM Exercise 5.

Using the CD-ROM

The accompanying CD-ROM allows the student to observe sessions, identify responses, and create responses for a variety of groups.

In CD-ROM Exercises 1 and 2, the student *creates a counselor response with a different focus* than the one given by the counselor. The student can compare the student-created response with other possibilities. Exercise 1 has eight responses to create, Exercise 2 has 1.

In CD-ROM Exercises 3 and 4, the student selects an appropriate response, intent, and focus, then *creates* a counselor response, and *compares* this student-created response to the actual counselor response. Exercise 3 has 28 selections and Exercise 4 has 10.

In CD-ROM Exercise 5, the student does the reverse of CD-ROM Exercises 3 and 4: the student *creates* a counselor response, then *identifies* the response, intent, and focus. The student then *compares* what has been created and identified with the actual counselor response. Exercise 5 has ten identifications.

The system requirements for using the CD-ROM are on the inside cover of this worktext. After inserting the CD-ROM in the computer, click on the BCRG icon to start the introduction to the CD-ROM. At any time, the introduction can be skipped by clicking anywhere on the screen. To repeat the introduction, click on the screen and then click the "replay intro" button.

The CD-ROM is organized as follows:

- Click S, Select, to choose Exercises 1–5. Clicking on "describe" will give a description of the selected group. Exercise numbers correspond to group numbers. Buttons will light up when appropriate.
- Click O, Observe group, to watch the selected group (1–5); the sessions can be observed with or without the response, intent, and focus identified by clicking the show/hide buttons.
- Click E, Do exercise, to begin or continue the selected group exercise. On this screen, click "proceed" to start. A note box can be opened to record questions or process comments or to state a rationale for a chosen response or identification. Notes and exercise work can be printed and saved by clicking "save work."
- Click V, View examples, to view examples of each basic counseling response, intent, and focus.
- Click H, Help, for detailed instructions for using the CD-ROM. "Overview" and "more help" are choices on this screen.
- Click Q, Quit, to exit at any time. The CD-ROM will close when "exit" is clicked.
- Click WEB to access the Web site.

In CD-ROM Exercises 1 and 2, the video will stop after selected counselor responses. The video will stop after *each part* of a multiple counselor response. The verbatim of the response and the response, intent, and focus will be shown. The student clicks "create" and keyboards a counselor response that has a different focus than the one given by the counselor. The student can compare the changed response to other given possibilities by clicking "compare." Because only clips of groups 1 and 2 are shown on the CD-ROM, students may want to watch these groups in their entirety on the videocassette.

In CD-ROM Exercises 3 and 4, the student selects a response, intent, and focus and then creates a response by clicking "create." The student must choose *who* and *what* in the focus box; *where* and *when* are optional. The student-created response, and the selected response, intent, and focus can be compared to the actual response that will play when "compare" is clicked.

In CD-ROM Exercise 5, the student creates a response and then identifies the response, intents, and focus. The student must choose *who* and *what* in the focus box; *where* and *when* are optional. The student-created response and the identified response, intent, and focus can be compared to the actual response that will play when "compare" is clicked.

Since student-created responses are requested in CD-ROM Exercises 3, 4, and 5, appropriateness can be discerned through supervision.

The CD-ROM help file is printed in Appendix C.

Accessing the Web Site

The CD-ROM is used to access the *Basic Counseling Responses in Groups* Web site. The WEB button is on every screen. See the troubleshooting file, Appendix C, for access problems.

Exercises for the Videocassette

There are two exercises for the videocassette in the worktext. They correspond to groups 1 and 2, respectively, on the videocassette. Each exercise requires that the students identify the RESPONSE, intent, and focus of selected counselor interactions. These selections are numbered and boxed in the transcripts included in the exercises. Identifications are not included in the selections. Suggested identifications for the selections follow the transcripts. Identifications can be done for counselor responses other than those selected by not looking at the transcript. The first number is the group number (*1*.7), followed by a lowercase letter if there are multiple sessions (1*b*.5). This group number is followed by the number of the client or counselor response (2.*14*). Multiple counselor responses are differentiated by lowercase letters (2.300*a* and 2.300*b*). In the transcripts for Groups 1 and 2, a CD-ROM icon with an up-arrow ⬆ is used at the beginning of clips, and a CD-ROM icon with a down-arrow ⬇ is used at the end of clips.

In the videocassette exercises, the identification of responses, intents, and focuses can be done using the Counseling Response Identification Format (CRIF) for Videocassette Exercises in Appendix A and on the CD-ROM in the forms folder. This format can be torn out and duplicated, set up as a template in a word-processing program, or downloaded as a template from the CD-ROM. The CRIF for Advanced Exercises 1–5 is also in Appendix A and can be downloaded from the CD-ROM. The sample CRIF on the next page is for the first response, Exercise 1. A second option is to write in the respective RESPONSE, intent, and focus on the transcript in the worktext. Selected interactions are boxed and spaces are provided with the respective response, intent, and focus icons (■ ● ▼). (See 1a.1, page 64.) Another option is to make a list of identifications rather than using a form; for example, 1a.1: Opening to acknowledge group experience.

Basic Counseling Responses in Groups

Counseling Response Indentification Format (CRIF)
for
Videocassette Exercises 1 and 2

Student **Sample** Counselor response **1a.1**

■ Response	● Intent	▼ Focus
☑ Opening or closing ☐ Attending ☐ Empathizing ☐ Paraphrasing ☐ Giving feedback ☐ Questioning ☐ Clarifying ☐ Directing ☐ Playing a hunch ☐ Noting a theme ☐ Noting a discrepancy ☐ Noting a connection ☐ Reframing ☐ Allowing silence ☐ Self-disclosing	☑ Acknowledge ☐ Explore ☐ Challenge ⇦ Check a response; For multiple or combination responses, number each response. ⇨ There can be multiple "whats." ⇨ One or both additives are in addition to a "who" or "what."	*Who* ☑ Group ☐ Subgroup ☐ Individual *What* ☑ Experience ☐ Thought ☐ Feeling ☐ Behavior Additives (optional) *Where* ☐ Context *When* ☐ Immediacy

Videocassette Exercise 1

Group 1/Women, Sessions, a, b, and c

- Suggested Identifications, page 82
- Diagram of group, Appendix A
- 16 identifications (including multiple responses)
- Transcript of Group 1/women follows

Observe

View Group 1/women, sessions 1a, 1b, and 1c on the videocassette.

Identify

Watch Group 1/women again. Stop the videocassette after each of the following selected counselor responses:

Session a: 1a.30 1a.35 1a.37 1a.45a + 45b 1a.59 1a.66

Session b: 1b.18 1b.42a + 42b 1b.49a, 49b + 49c 1b.51 1b.63

Session c: 1c.18

Using the CRIF format (Appendix A and CD-ROM), the blanks in the following transcript, or a list, identify the RESPONSE, intent, and focus for each of the selected counselor responses. An example is given for the first identification.

Compare

Check Suggested Identifications, Exercise 1, to compare identified RESPONSES, intents, and focuses.

Reflect

1. Discuss the development of this group from sessions a through c. Note the use of "we," especially in session c.
2. Discuss the gender and diversity variables evidenced in this group. How are they addressed in the group? Did the counselor need to do something different? Note especially 1b.68–74.
3. How do you think the counselor handled Barbara's anger that was directed toward her? How would you handle it differently?
4. See counselor responses 1a.35 and 1a.37; 1b.49c and 1b.51. What is the purpose of using the one-two punch response, and how does it affect the group?
5. See client response 1b.57. Identify the counseling RESPONSE, intent, and focus.
6. Session c, the final session of Group 1/women, ends with the counselor asking "How is this ending like other endings in your life?" If you were a member of this group, how would you answer this question?

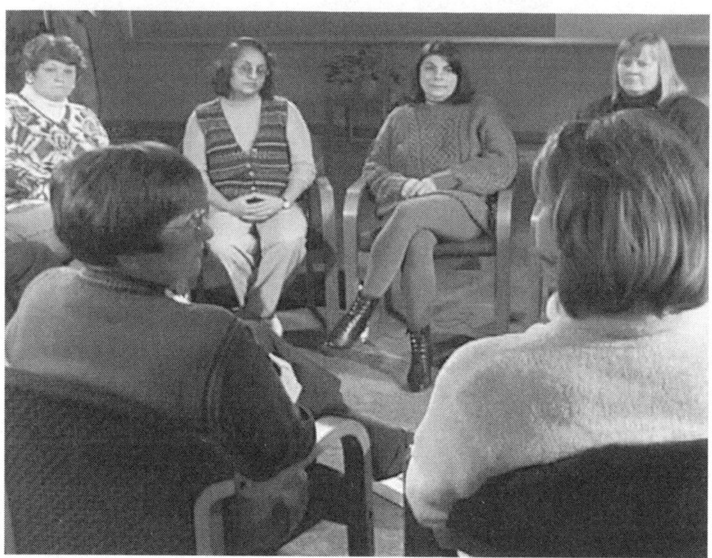

GROUP 1/WOMEN, SESSION A

la. 1	COUNSELOR	"So where would the group like to start today?" OPENING to acknowledge group experience
la. 2	SUE	"I'm here today because I'm kinda in a crossroad of my life . . ."
la. 3	COUNSELOR	"And your name is?" *Noncounseling response*
la. 4	SUE	"Oh, my name is Sue, . . . my daught . . . my last child has left my house. And, . . . so I don't think I have empty nest syndrome, because it's really wonderful that she's gone, but I still feel that . . . I'm changing roles and I wanted to just be around other women and see if anyone's experienced it, and . . . to get some support about what's gonna, you know, what's lying ahead of me."
la. 5	COUNSELOR	"Um-hmm." ATTENDING to acknowledge individual experience
la. 6	LINDA	"My name is Linda, and I have similar concerns with Sue, . . . I have . . . two children . . . 21 and 18 and I 'm struggling with making the transition from being the parent of a teenager to the parent of an adult child. And I thought it would be helpful to talk to some other people about how they made that, made that change."
la. 7	DOROTHY	"This is a little hard for me to listen to because I have three stepsons. All who are of the age to be grown up and out of their homes, but they are in California. And they've made poor choices in their lives, and one of them particularly continues to make poor choices and . . . only one has a high school diploma, they're really

		wrestling with, how to make their future bright, and it's because they have not become an adult yet. They're still children. I do have a granddaughter who is up in this area, . . . and she doesn't have a father that's fully functioning in her life and it's really a, a, sad thing, so I'm, I'm, hoping someday that'll all change and we'll have great kids also. So far that's not the way it's worked out; it's been very challenging."
1a. 8	COUNSELOR	"So what's it's like to hear some of the group talk about being joyful around us?" QUESTIONING to explore individual experience
1a. 9	DOROTHY	"It's very sad. . . . the last time, and the oldest son . . . The last time I talked to him was a, he was in a great deal of need and . . . we have taken a stand that we're not going to continue to provide, and rescue and enable and we could be there again. And, . . . may even die, . . . I don't like to say that out loud but . . ."
1a. 10	COUNSELOR	"You're really not sure he'll make it." PARAPHRASING to acknowledge individual experience
1a. 11	DOROTHY	"I'm not sure he'll make it. Um-hmm."
1a. 12	LINDA	"I really identify with what you are saying, . . . about . . . how difficult it is to watch children make their choices, and my children are younger, but I think that's part of the . . . issue that I'm working with in transition, and that is how do you . . ."
1a. 13	COUNSELOR	"How do 'I'?" DIRECTING to challenge individual behavior
1a. 14	LINDA	"Yeah. How do I let them, not let them, how do I adjust to their making their own choices?"
1a. 15a 1a. 15b	COUNSELOR	"I'd like to get back to what you were talking about a little bit Dorothy, in terms of listening to others around their joy and really getting in touch with your pain and actual fear that, your older son, stepson, could actually not make it, die, in the process of trying to find himself. DIRECTING to challenge individual behavior *The counselor is actually directing the group back to what an individual has just said.* "What's that like to share that with folks here?" QUESTIONING to challenge individual experience in context
1a. 16	DOROTHY	"Um, tsk, . . ."
1a. 17	COUNSELOR	"It's OK . . ." *Not a counseling response*

1a. 18	DOROTHY	"It's like something . . . I don't think I'll ever experience."
1a. 19	COUNSELOR	"Their joy?" CLARIFYING to explore individual feeling
1a. 20	DOROTHY	"Uh-huh."
1a. 21	COUNSELOR	"Uh-huh. So in the group you end up feeling . . ." QUESTIONING to challenge individual feeling in context
1a. 22	DOROTHY	"Lonely."
1a. 23	COUNSELOR	"Lonely, yeah." EMPATHIZING to acknowledge individual feeling
1a. 24	DOROTHY	"And that my husband and I didn't do a good enough job. Part of it's feeling like geez, did I do something wrong? Was I not a good enough, I was the stick-it, I was the stick-it? I was the wicked stepmother, and yet all that we did we wonder if still could we have done more? Could we have done something differently? Could we have said something differently? . . . I know, as we sit and talk about this, I'm wondering now if it's not part of what feeds into why I give so much to other people. Because I wonder did I not give enough to the two, the three that were closest to us . . . I never got that connection before."
1a. 25	LINDA	"I wonder if guilt is uniquely a female phenomenon?"
1a. 26	DOROTHY	"Maybe, I don't know."
1a. 27	LINDA	"Most mothers I know feel guilty."
1a. 28	VEE	"As I sat here and listened to you Dorothy, I kind of made a switch. I know I came in with a concern that was mine. But, for a moment I was transported into . . . my mother's shoes, and the choices her son made—my brother. And I'm just sitting here feeling somewhat your fear. Thank you for saying what you said because that, that's helped me."
1a. 29	DOROTHY	"Thank you." (deep sigh)
1a. 30	COUNSELOR	"There seems to be sadness in the group . . . joining you right now." ■ ____________ ● ____________ ▼ ____________
1a. 31	LYNN	"It is absolutely amazing to me how quickly in a group situation my buttons can get pushed like this. As you're talking, I'm at that same faith, I feel really guilty, and I know where it comes from. I mean it sounds like I'm not unique in this at all . . . but my nephew is in jail. And his . . . my sister struggles with her life tremendously, always has. She's . . . an alcoholic and has been in and out of treatment a lot, and . . . has now had to leave her family completely and

		go to another state and just concentrate on being sober. I mean she's almost died many times and, . . . when we grew up, in growing up, my, she's my stepsister, and, . . . her father left her and my mom, deserted them when they were young, she never really knew her dad. And then, my dad came along and, they got married and he would do the bringing her presents and all that kind of stuff. She was like five years old. Then I was born and all that stopped, she wasn't his kid, she, he didn't have anything to do with her, and I was his. I was the first born. And so there was this tremendous resentment, all our lives for my not being, . . . my being the spoiled one. And then, she grows up, becomes an alcoholic, has all these terrible problems, her children run away from home, her son's in jail, all of her four grandchildren are in foster care. I marry a wonderful man, I have four healthy children, and my mother is very attentive to my sister because of her problems, and I'm just kind of, I feel neglected. I feel lonely. I feel out of it. Because I don't have enough problems. I look for problems to be able to say, here's me, and so you're talking, and I immediately felt lonely. And selfish. Because it's like, I'm here, I'm here, everybody see me and I, I absolutely hate that, and, and I'm hoping that some day I'll grow past that so I can deal with that and not have that, immediately feel so . . . I don't like that in me at all, it makes me a little ashamed. I feel so ashamed."
1a. 32	VEE	"As I'm sitting here, I can feel my temples, and I can feel the need to take deep breaths. And I know I'm still not past what you've shared with us, and I still feel the need . . . to either go beyond, and spend more time on it, maybe dwell on it more, and I really haven't, I feel I need to hear from you too. Because it seemed like you started the ball rolling with what, where you were at. And, then Dorothy shared, and I never heard back from you, I feel I need to do that. I need to hear from where you're at. What, are concerns."
1a. 33	SUE	"What Dorothy said triggered . . . a really deep pain in my heart. . . . my daughter's leaving home, is really a wonderful, wonderful thing for us . . . because we had a child die seven years ago. And, . . . he was a troubled kid and, . . . he did drugs, and he dropped out of school and, . . . we had to ask him to leave our home. And . . . he left our home and then he . . . straightened up, he graduated top of his class in California and he came home a changed person. And one night he did something very stupid, and . . . he was in a car crash and he died. And he never got the chance to leave home. And so I don't know if her leaving home, . . . it's hard to let her go. . . . because I don't want to lose another one, and so when you talk about kids not being perfect, . . . I loved him with all my heart, even though he wasn't perfect. And, so when you tell me, I can share your fear. It is so scary and you feel so out of control. So, I guess I was holding back a little."

la. 34	DOROTHY	"You, you've already experienced what I'm fearful is going to happen. You've come through it."
la. 35	COUNSELOR	"So, what's it like to hear your greatest fear happening?" ■ ______ ● ______ ▼ ______
la. 36	DOROTHY	"Oh, I'll get through that too. I mean, she looks like she got through it somehow. I'm sure it's still there, I'm sure that it never goes away."
la. 37	COUNSELOR	"Where is the rest of the group with this pain?" ■ ______ ● ______ ▼ ______
la. 38	JEAN	"Right there in it too. If not, if not having experienced the same kind of pain, just, that that kind that could happen, and, I can, the thought of losing a child, it's not how its supposed to be. It hurts, I'm hurting."
la. 39 ⬇	LINDA	"I resonate with the guilt that I hear and . . . trying to figure out for myself how you deal with some of that guilt and . . . one of the ways I think that I dealt with it . . . is by accepting a notion of free will. Somehow I think that . . . as a mother and as I heard other mothers talk, we feel as if we should be able to control the world. Or at least our children's world. And control their decisions and control what happens to them. . . . but once I accepted the notion of free will, I understood that, at least for myself, no matter what I want, or no matter what I think, that my children have the ability to make decisions that are outside the realm of what I can control. . . ."
la. 40	COUNSELOR	"So Linda, what's it like to hear her pain." QUESTIONING to explore individual feeling
la. 41	LINDA	". . . It makes me angry. Because . . . I think it's unfair to . . . put all of that burden on mothers."
la. 42	COUNSELOR	"Um-hmm, to not have that control." PLAYING A HUNCH to challenge individual behavior
la. 43 ⬆	LINDA	"No, I think it's unfair that we've been socialized to believe that we do when we don't, and that creates guilt. It's anger I think."
la. 44	SUE	"I can relate to what you are saying Linda, because I think we have been told and we have been raised to believe that we have more control than what we really have over our children and the world and other people. I do believe that there is the thing called free will and I do believe people make choices, and I do believe that stuff just happens and I think that's what's helped me come to the place knowing that my son had free will, and that night he had free will. He's the one that was driving his car 80 miles an hour. And it's knowing that, if I would have had the choice that night, I wouldn't have chosen that. And that is what has helped me even though I

		still am sad, and I have lost . . . I know that if I would have had that choice I wouldn't have made it. And there is free will, I do believe that, and the control that we have I don't think we have anywhere near as much control as we think we have. I think we've been fed a big line."
1a. 45a 1a. 4ba	COUNSELOR	"I noticed there is a real shift in the energy in this group from sadness to anger, to sort of wanting to take hold and . . . So where are we now in this group?" ■ ______________ ● ______________ ▼ ______________
1a. 46	LYNN	"I feel real distant."
1a. 47	COUNSELOR	"You're feeling distant." EMPATHIZING to acknowledge individual feeling
1a. 48	LYNN	"The more the group talked, the more I felt myself just kinda numbing to it. And . . . I don't even know how to describe the emotion that I have right now, my heart's beating really fast and . . . it's almost like I'm angry and I don't even know what I'm angry at. I feel real distant. I, I, don't feel the empathy that I feel like I should feel. And, I feel angry. I think it's anger, I don't know."
1a. 49	SUE	"Are you scared because . . . things are going, are OK, with your . . ."
1a. 50	LYNN	"No, I'm not thinking about my children, I'm thinking about me."
1a. 51	SUE	"Oh."
1a. 52	LYNN	"See, it's like, it's almost, I don't . . ."
1a. 53	COUNSELOR	"What about you Lynn?" QUESTIONING to challenge individual experience
1a. 54	LYNN	". . . I'm inadequate, I'm not enough, . . ."
1a. 55	COUNSELOR	"In this group?" QUESTIONING to challenge individual experience in context
1a. 56	LYNN	"Yeah, yeah, I, don't even know if this is rational."
1a. 57	COUNSELOR	"Uh-huh, Just stay with it." DIRECTING to challenge individual behavior
1a. 58	LYNN	"Yeah it's . . . I've never lost a child, I've never . . . and even as I say that, that just, I hate that, I mean I hate that I would think like that."
1a. 59	COUNSELOR	"To belong to this group you would have to have lost a child." ■ ______________ ● ______________ ▼ ______________
1a. 60	LYNN	"Or be able to just feel, not feel for myself, in this group, just be feeling for others, who are feeling painful and I'm feeling selfish. I'm thinking, I don't know, I feel embarrassed, I feel ashamed, that

		“I still have such selfish feelings and I’ve worked so hard not to be here and I’m still here. And I feel even talking about it is, like, is this real, or am I talking about it, so you’re all looking at me now, and I don’t want attention even. At the same time, you know what, I, it’s hard for me to describe it but I don’t like the place that I’m at. And so I didn’t feel when everybody was, and I did to, it’s hard to describe it. I don’t like it. I can tell you that.”
1a. 61	COUNSELOR	“Is there room enough in this group for you to not feel what others are feeling?” QUESTIONING to challenge individual feeling in context
1a. 62	LYNN	“Yeah, I just don’t like it.”
1a. 63	COUNSELOR	“Um-hmm.” ATTENDING to acknowledge individual experience
1a. 64	LYNN	“It’s just not a comfortable place.”
1a. 65	DOROTHY	“As I listen to you talk, I, I think maybe the gift you have for this group for me is that, I need to learn how to be more selfish, and I can’t learn it from people who aren’t already selfish . . . so I think I’m gonna learn a lot from you in this group.”
1a. 66	COUNSELOR	“So what happens when Dorothy says you’re gonna teach her about being selfish?” ■ ______________ ● ______________ ▼ ______________
1a. 67	LYNN	“It’s a real conflict. I mean it’s a tremendous conflict, it’s like I’m working all my life not to be selfish. It’s just, and she just said she had the image of me being selfish.”
1a. 68	LINDA	“But maybe you’re using the term *selfish* comes across to me in many ways like guilt, I’m gonna talk about that. Guilt that . . .”
1a. 69	LYNN	“What I meant by *selfish,* I still think I’m, I’m still, I don’t want to be so self absorbed where in a situation that isn’t about me, I can let go of me and be just with the person that is struggling with whatever they’re struggling with. And it just seems like I just carry me in whatever situation I’m in too much.”
1a. 70	SUE	“I mean I don’t want anybody to have what happened to me. It’s, I’m happy that you have a good life, that that you have four kids, and you have a husband, and that’s wonderful.”
1a. 71	LYNN	“This is weird, because you’re comforting me. Isn’t that weird?”
1a. 72	COUNSELOR	“What’s weird about it?” QUESTIONING to challenge individual feeling
1a. 73	LYNN	“I feel really embarrassed, I wish I could take it away, I wish could go back about half an hour and not have said anything. ’cause I feel ya know, I feel . . . I feel so guilty.”

1a. 74	BARBARA	"You know, you keep saying, you keep saying that it's weird, but you keep talking about it."
1a. 75	LYNN	"I know, I know, I think well who, who brought it up, I did. I'm the one that said it. I brought the attention to myself."
1a. 76	BARBARA	"So why do you do that? Why do you think its weird? So why do you talk about it?"
1a. 77	LYNN	"I'm wondering now if that's the kind of person I am, if I do that too much. If I bring attention to myself too much."
1a. 78	COUNSELOR	"We are getting close to ending today, how would the group like to close? Kind of shifting gears here." CLOSING to acknowledge group experience
1a. 79	JEAN	"I, I just want to know for Lynn how is it gonna to be if we end right now?"
1a. 80	LYNN	"I'm real ready for it to end, that would be fine. I'm ready for a new day now, and a new place."

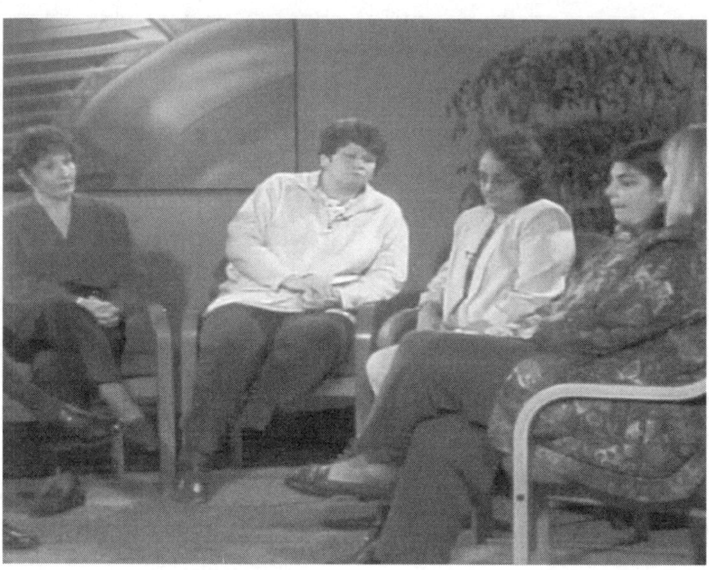

GROUP 1/WOMEN, SESSION B

1b. 1a 1b. 1b	COUNSELOR	"So where would the group like to start today?" OPENING to acknowledge group experience (The group is silent) ALLOWING SILENCE to acknowledge group experience
1b. 2	LINDA	"One of the things that stuck with me as I thought about many of the things that Lynn said . . . was the sense of . . . how painful, I want to say undeserved, but a sense of undeserved love can be. As a middle child I had an older sister that was my father's favorite. And I always thought that would be such a neat place to be in, you know, either the oldest so that you're the favorite, or the youngest so that you get all that special attention, and I guess I never thought about the fact that it could be painful for the person who's on the receiving end of that. I just always saw that as something so wonderful, I only saw the up side of it, and I think I see what you helped me see was there's a down side to that."
1b. 3	COUNSELOR	"So your family is in this room." PLAYING A HUNCH to challenge individual experience
1b. 4	LINDA	"Yeah, what looks like selfishness is really empathy, empathy for that other person, hurting for that other person, . . . feeling for that other person."
1b. 5	COUNSELOR	"Where are others in the group today?" QUESTIONING to challenge group experience

1b. 6	BARBARA	"Well, this is really hard for me, but . . . I was . . . I had a really bad week last week . . . it kinda has to do with being selfish. Because I was thinking, I was a little bit angry that nobody wanted to, that I came in with a certain thing to do and it's like it went in a different direction, and it was very frustrating and so I got angry and this is very embarrassing to tell everybody because that to me is being very, very selfish. Again I want the whole group to work on my problem. Not to do what they're doing."
1b. 7	COUNSELOR	"So who were you feeling angry with, Barbara?" QUESTIONING to challenge individual feeling
1b. 8	BARBARA	"Eventually myself, for feeling that way."
1b. 9	COUNSELOR	"How about here in the group?" QUESTIONING to challenge individual feeling in context
1b. 10	BARBARA	"Nobody in particular, but it's very uncomfortable for me to have had that thought."
1b. 11	COUNSELOR	"Uh-huh, I wonder if you could. I'm sorry." *Incomplete response*
1b. 12	LYNN	"I was just gonna ask what you would have liked from us? What could we have given you?"
1b. 13	BARBARA	"I don't know. I just . . . Yeah, I don't know."
1b. 14	COUNSELOR	"I wonder if you could stay with the anger? I think that's important." DIRECTING to challenge individual feeling *This is DIRECTING, but in the form of a question.*
1b. 15	BARBARA	"Staying angry is very hard for me."
1b. 16	COUNSELOR	"Uh-huh. So I'm encouraging you to kinda push yourself a bit and with us here in this room if that's where you're feeling it." DIRECTING to challenge individual feeling *Note that the context is "room," not group.*
1b. 17	BARBARA	"The minute that I get angry . . . it's gone. I mean, I have a, I'm sure that everybody's had a really crappy childhood too. I had a really crappy childhood and both alcoholic parents, and two very bad marriages, and through all that, I just figured it was all my fault. I think that I've come a long way in understanding that it's not my fault, but I still can't get past this being afraid of anger. I've never been angry with any of the people that did any of the things to me."
1.b. 18	COUNSELOR	"Uh-huh, But you did feel anger when you left here?" ■ ________________ ● ________________ ▼ ________________

1b. 19	BARBARA	"Yeah, it's safe for me to feel anger by myself."
1b. 20	COUNSELOR	"Right. And so I wonder if there's a way for you to begin to notice who you might feel that with here?" QUESTIONING to challenge individual feeling in context
1b. 21	BARBARA	"Well, you keep asking me that, I'm beginning to feel that with you, because I don't feel angry with a single person."
1b. 22	COUNSELOR	"Except right now." NOTING A DISCREPANCY to challenge individual feeling with immediacy
1b. 23	BARBARA	"Because you're pushing me."
1b. 24	COUNSELOR	"Uh-huh . . . what's it like, what are you feeling, what's happening?" QUESTIONING to challenge individual feeling
1b. 25	BARBARA	"It's shame."
1b. 26	COUNSELOR	"What might happen?" QUESTIONING to challenge individual behavior
1b. 27	BARBARA	"Well, what's gonna happen is I'm gonna back down and I'm just gonna sit here and be quiet probably."
1b. 28	COUNSELOR	"See if you can stay with it . . ." DIRECTING to challenge individual behavior
1b. 29	BARBARA	"I think it's gone now."
1b. 30	COUNSELOR	"How's the group right now with this?" QUESTIONING to challenge group feeling with immediacy
1b. 31	SUE	"I'm gettin' kinda mad at you too . . ."
1b. 32	COUNSELOR	"Uh-huh . . . What's happening for you Sue?" QUESTIONING to challenge individual feeling
1b. 33	SUE	"Well, I'm just, I'm just, I'm just watching you push her, and push her and I think you're making her feel worse and worse. I don't want to see her feel worse and worse . . ."
1b. 34	COUNSELOR	"So you're feeling protective of Barbara?" PLAYING A HUNCH to challenge individual feeling *In question form*
1b. 35	SUE	"Yeah."
1b. 36	COUNSELOR	"Um-hmm. So that she can't have her anger?" PLAYING A HUNCH to challenge individual feeling *In question form*

1b. 37	SUE	"She, she can be angry, but I don't want her to hurt."
1b. 38	LYNN	"I don't want her to lose her anger, I want us to be safe enough to be really angry. That's why I asked what you want from us. I want to know what you didn't get, I want you to feel angry, I want this to be safe enough where you can feel angry and discover nobody is going to die here."
1b. 39	BARBARA	"Well I know, I mean I've done, I've done a lot of work around this and I can't get angry. I can't. It's like I physically stop myself."
1b. 40	COUNSELOR	"You didn't." GIVING FEEDBACK to challenge individual feeling
1b. 41	BARBARA	"I know. I don't know how to do it."
1b. 42a 1b. 42b	COUNSELOR	"I'm confused because you did get angry, you did show some anger, it was momentary, it was fleeting, but you had it, it was here, so you can." ■ ______________ ● ______________ ▼ ______________ "Where's the rest of the group now?"
1b. 43	JEAN	"I'm struggling with wanting to do this but knowing, but knowing it's like right here and it's not going down that I'm angry at you. For putting this out here and I don't know what it's about. And so I'm angry that something happened and I didn't pick up on it. And that I didn't ask you, but then more than angry at me I'm angry at you, 'cause I don't know what it is as Lynn asked that you're wanting and needing and, and, it went down for awhile when you were talking but know it's back up about . . . before I experienced you being able to talk and express your feelings and so I'm angry that all of a sudden you couldn't, and what happened."
1b. 44	BARBARA	"Actually, I thought I was. It's very frustrating for me not to be able to feel angry. And I brought it up because everybody was talking about how they felt, so I was just trying to share what my week was like and what happened so, and you know, I would love to be able to explain it, but I can't."
1b. 45	LINDA	"I resonate with some of the things you are saying about anger, what I hear is that you can be angry, you can be angry with yourself, very well, and you probably do that very well."
1b. 46	BARBARA	"Yeah I do."
1b. 47	LINDA	"But . . . I also had an experience of violence in my life, it was a cousin that I loved very much who married a man that was very violent that I know that fear of what happens when anger gets out of control. And . . . so I really resonate as I listen to you talk, I think I, I think I understand what you're saying. And I can hear other people saying, 'Tell us more; help us understand.' But I think

		I understand what you're saying, that not wanting to have conflict because if it begins to happen it may escalate in ways that you can no longer control. So I think, at least I feel like I hear what you are saying even though you're not saying the words."
1b. 48	BARBARA	"I had two incidents in my life and they were both with the husband, that I got so angry that I sorta lost what I was doing. One I jumped out of a moving car. And the other one, I just broke a shower. I just shattered a glass shower I was so angry. It terrified me."
1b. 49a 1b. 49b 1b. 49c	COUNSELOR	"I wonder if others struggle with that?" ■ ____________ ● ____________ ▼ ____________ "Some are nodding your heads." ■ ____________ ● ____________ ▼ ____________ "So, Barbara, how are you feeling sharing all this with the group today?" ■ ____________ ● ____________ ▼ ____________
1b. 50	BARBARA	"I actually feel pretty good about it, I . . . I just think that we all live with a lot of secrets. And . . . it's not going to do me any good to keep a secret here because the point of being here is work on the stuff that's hard for ya. So it's hard for me to say it, but I'm glad I did."
1b. 51	COUNSELOR	"So how does the group feel about what Barbara just said? What she did today?" ■ ____________ ● ____________ ▼ ____________
1b. 52	LYNN	"Wow, in the first group we had I felt so naked. And now I really feel more a sense of connection with the group and even as we're talking about struggles with anger, I'm hearing us all talk about, I don't feel so separate, I feel part of the group. And a lot of the areas that I felt alone, I don't feel so alone."
1b. 53	DOROTHY	"I think as coming out of our culture, culture has such an attitude that anger is destructive and has so many negative things that I know even in this group we've tenderly gone, well maybe not tenderly, but gingerly have gone there hesitatingly and . . . and that's a hard thing to do, without getting angry."
1b. 54	LINDA	"You mentioned culture and I think that . . . coming from a different cultural perspective I probably have a different perspective on anger, its easier for me . . . and I wonder how much of that is just having a different cultural experience?"
1b. 55	BARBARA	"I think it probably has a lot to do with it."
1b. 56a 1b. 56b	COUNSELOR	"Still feeling a lot." EMPATHIZING to acknowledge individual feeling

1b. 56c		"Your eyes are still teary." GIVING FEEDBACK to acknowledge individual behavior "How about the rest of you?" QUESTIONING to challenge group experience
1b. 57	VEE	"Well I get the sense that you are expressing your anger except you're crying. And it seems like that's how you . . . show your anger. And control it, and manage it, and I think if you were to allow yourself to say I am feeling anger except this is the way I show it. I don't know how that would sit with you."
1b. 58	BARBARA	"Well, no, I've said that. I mean I know that's the way I express it."
1b. 59	COUNSELOR	"So you're talking about tears being part of an expression of anger." PARAPHRASING to acknowledge individual behavior
1b. 60	VEE	"Yeah, and it seems like women would find it easier to take that route and . . . speaking for myself and from a cultural perspective, it's a little different. I don't always feel that it's necessary to express anger and . . . and if you can recognize that you're angry you can express it any way you want to, you don't have to have prescribed ways of expressing that feeling. I feel that as a woman I need to recognize that and not feel I'm bound by society telling me how, where, and why, I should express my emotions."
1b. 61	COUNSELOR	"And are you saying as a woman coming from a different culture it's a different, it's different or are you saying as a woman I should be able to express my . . . ?" QUESTIONING to challenge individual feeling
1b. 62	VEE	"A little bit of both. A little bit of both."
1b. 63	COUNSELOR	"Uh-huh, and I'm wondering if that's some of what you are talking about too, Linda, in terms of I don't know that I have trouble with anger in the same way that people do here." ■ ____________ ● ____________ ▼ ____________
1b. 64	LINDA	"Um-hmm, yeah, and I heard some of that coming out in Vee's voice as she was talking, I heard a comfortableness with anger that's different from what I heard . . . Dorothy talking about which was an uncomfortableness with anger . . . and I guess I'm feeling some anger for Barbara because she brought something to us and said you guys aren't dealing with my stuff and we kinda didn't deal with her stuff and so I'm thinking why aren't we dealing with her stuff so I kinda got angry for her since she wasn't able to get angry for herself."
1b. 65	BARBARA	"So how do you do it?"
1b. 66	LINDA	"Well I was thinking . . . I probably should answer a question. I wasn't thinking about it. I should probably answer your question. I think it's a, a feeling when things are not fair that that's not right."

1b. 67	BARBARA	"But I have those feelings, I just. I just don't get . . ."
1b. 68	LINDA	"But I think I'd live in a world where things are not fair a lot and you experience it a lot and so you don't get angry every time, but because the experience is so frequent you tend to exhibit anger more than other people would be able to understand because it isn't just the one incident. It's not that you're not angry—probably at other things—it's just that you can't suppress the anger all the time because it happens too frequently in a way that I think is very difficult for people who don't experience that as a constant daily situation can understand."
1b. 69	COUNSELOR	"I, I wonder if it's happened here? In this group?" QUESTIONING to challenge individual experience in context
1b. 70	LINDA	"Not so much in this group . . ."
1b. 71	COUNSELOR	"Would you tell us if it did?" QUESTIONING to challenge individual behavior
1b. 72	LINDA	"Oh yes."
1b. 73	VEE	"I was wondering that same thing too."
1b. 74	LINDA	"Yeah. I would. I've tried to become good at telling people when it does but that's why I think I wanted to be angry for Barbara because I thought—I have a competency here—that I want her to say I'm really angry you guys didn't deal with my stuff and be upfront about it."

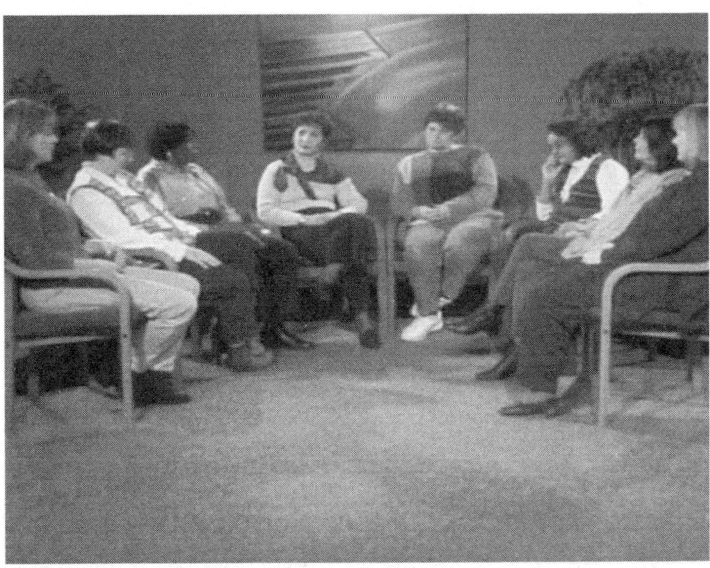

GROUP 1/WOMEN, SESSION C

1c. 1	COUNSELOR	"I wonder where the group is around the sense of not being good enough. Like that came up around parenting being mothers' issues, and it came up here in the group." QUESTIONING to challenge group feeling
1c. 2	BARBARA	"Well, I don't know. For me it's helpful to know that I'm certainly not out there all by myself feeling like I'm not good enough. And I really think this has been a terrific . . . lesson not only in not feeling good enough but also discussing anger and knowing that it is actually shared."
1c. 3	COUNSELOR	"You're not alone." EMPATHIZING to acknowledge individual feeling
1c. 4	BARBARA	"And shared by everybody."
1c. 5	COUNSELOR	"It was kind of universal wasn't it?" ■ ____________ ● ____________ ▼ ____________
1c. 6	LYNN	"I think I don't remember who said it in one of our groups, we talked about the question good enough. Good enough for what? You know? That really stuck with me. Good enough for what? Good enough to be a human, I'm good enough to be of value to others, profitable you know, and put up with others. The question itself is wrong. Good enough for what?"
1c. 7	JEAN	"And I know myself that that question will come up throughout any new thing, any other thing that I'm uncomfortable. I'll always wonder that, I'll always know that in this experience I did experience being good enough in here. There's so many other places that

		I don't ever feel that and that's the sadness I won't have that I will take it and cherish. I'll always question that but I know here I experienced being good enough."
1c. 8	SUE	"I guess I'd like to thank everybody for making it be a very safe place . . . I felt very safe every time we've been here. And . . . it's also helped me think about different things about myself and I've heard everybody phrase. I heard you talk about anger, and I've heard you talk about assertiveness and anger in different ways and allowed me to take another look at myself and that . . . maybe be a little more gentle with myself where anger is concerned. I want to thank you all for giving me that gift."
1c. 9	LINDA	"Sue said eloquently, I think, what I feel so I don't say this eloquently, but the . . . openess with which people shared things that were important to them also helped in me figuring out some things for myself."
1c. 10	LYNN	"You know, as we're experiencing a little silence, I remember at the very beginning silence was so awkward I wanted to jump in and fill it in. Seems like we've really gotten to a point where we can be comfortable with that it's OK if there's . . . silence is OK. I noticed that."
1c. 11	BARBARA	"I think, I think I'm struck by how comfortable I was comfortable. I don't know if I'm speaking for the group, but I think that we were all kind of . . . quick to get to trust each other and get to know each other and that kind of amazed me. I didn't think that would happen."
1c. 12	JEAN	"And, and then because of that I think it was hard work that we did that, and then when we really had to do some of the hard stuff in the group, for me that trust that I had experienced and that I think we all felt it was . . ."
1c. 13	COUNSELOR	"What was the hard stuff?" QUESTIONING to challenge individual experience
1c. 14	JEAN	"To do the hard stuff, and to deal with the angers and the other issues of being good enough, but because I felt trusted and that it was a 'we' and it wasn't just I, I felt safe in the 'we' here."
1c. 15	COUNSELOR	"So it managed to hang together even when we were pulling apart?" PARAPHRASING to acknowledge group experience *In question form*
1c. 16	SUE	"I wonder if anybody feels like we take 'we' with us when we leave this room?" *Note that this may be an example of a client making a counseling response: QUESTIONING to challenge group feeling.*
1c. 17	VEE	"I was just thinking there was a sense of sadness when we were trying to talk about where we were and how it had been, but as I kept hearing everyone talk it seemed like the goodbyes are not

		going to be final. There's going to be this wonderful image I can bring up of everybody here in the room and their strengths and their contributions and where I was when I first started and what I'm leaving with. Leaving with one special gift that I'd like to say I think if you hadn't started talking about anger the way you did I wouldn't have quite realized what my culture gave to me as a strength which I never really . . . recognized until you brought it up, so thank you."
1c. 18	COUNSELOR	"So I'm wondering how this is like other endings in your life? Our saying goodbye today." ■ ______________ ● ______________ ▼ ______________
1c. 19	BARBARA	"This is unlike any ending in my life because this is an ending where I'm feeling a lot of love and warmth for everybody and I don't usually end that way."
1c. 20	COUNSELOR	"Oh." ATTENDING to acknowledge individual experience
1c. 21	BARBARA	"Yeah."

Suggested Identifications for Selected Counselor Responses

Videocassette Exercise 1: Group 1/Women

Number	Response, Intent, Focus
1a. 30	EMPATHIZING to acknowledge group feeling with immediacy in context
1a. 35	QUESTIONING to challenge individual experience
1a. 37	QUESTIONING to challenge group experience *1a.35 + 1a.37 = one-two punch*
1a. 45a	GIVING FEEDBACK to acknowledge group feeling
1a. 45b	QUESTIONING to explore group experience with immediacy in context *Multiple response*
1a. 59	PLAYING A HUNCH to challenge individual experience in context
1a. 66	QUESTIONING to challenge individual experience
1b. 18	NOTING A DISCREPANCY to challenge individual feeling *Note the individual focus in the next several counselor responses.*
1b. 42a	NOTING A DISCREPANCY to challenge individual feeling in context
1b. 42b	QUESTIONING to challenge group experience with immediacy *Multiple response; note different focus*
1b. 49a	QUESTIONING to challenge group feelings
1b. 49b	GIVING FEEDBACK to acknowledge group behavior
1b. 49c	QUESTIONING to challenge individual feeling in context *Multiple response*
1b. 51	QUESTIONING to challenge group feeling and behavior *With 49c, an example of the one-two punch*
1b. 63	NOTING A CONNECTION to challenge subgroup feeling in context
1c. 18	QUESTIONING to challenge individual experience in context

Videocassette Exercise 2

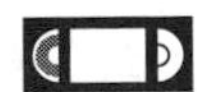

Group 2/Boys

- Suggested Identifications, page 117
- Diagram of group, Appendix A
- 12 identifications (including multiple responses)
- Transcript of Group 2/boys follows

Observe

View Group 2/boys on the videocassette.

Identify

Watch Group 2/boys again. Stop the videocassette after each of the following selected counselor responses:

2.8 | 2.30 | 2.40 | 2.75 | 2.169 | 2.223 | 2.298 | 2.334 | 2.344 | 2.445 | 2.554a + 2.554b

Using the CRIF format (Appendix A and CD-ROM), the blanks in the following transcript, or a list, identify the RESPONSE, intent, and focus for each of the selected counselor responses. An example is given for the first identification.

Compare

Check Suggested Identifications, Exercise 2, to compare identified RESPONSES, intents, and focuses.

Reflect

1. Discuss the development of this group. Include in the discussion how the behavior of individual members changes. Note the change in pronouns.
2. Discuss the family, cultural, and age variables that influence the group's development. Note especially 2.106.
3. What norms would you, as a counselor for this group, want the group to follow?
4. Discuss the therapeutic value of this group.
5. See counselor response 2.75. Note the reactions of the clients. How would you react to this question?
6. See client comment 2.341. Identify this as a counseling response.
7. See counselor responses 2.512, 2.523, 2.545, and 2.550. What do you think the counselor was trying to do with these responses?
8. See 2.558–2.568. If you were the counselor during this interaction, how would you respond?

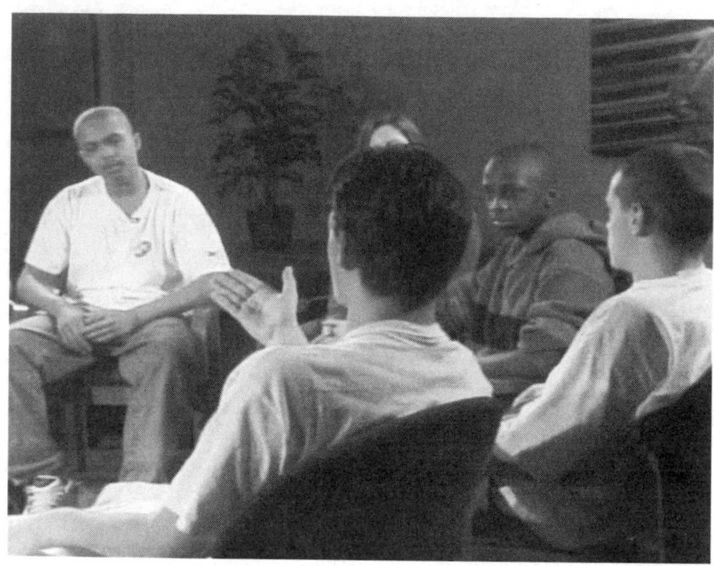

GROUP 2/BOYS

2. 1	COUNSELOR	"Where would the group like to start today?" OPENING to explore group experience
2. 2	THOMAS	"Hoops, where we were. Ha. I'd like to talk about where we were. Ha."
2. 3	WALLACE	"I think we should just start wherever."
2. 4	THOMAS	"Start, man, dude. Where?"
2. 5	ERIC	"Why don't you think of something, Jennifer?"
2. 6	WALLACE	"Yeah, Jennifer."
2. 7	THOMAS	"Yeah, you're the one's 'spose to run this thing." *Note this challenge to the role of the counselor.*
2. 8	COUNSELOR	"It seems like the group is feeling nervous. Not knowing where to begin?" ■ ______________ ● ______________ ▼ ______________
2. 9	THOMAS	"Nervous? I'm a . . ."
2. 10	ERIC	"We can talk about school."
2. 11	THOMAS	"I'm just waiting for someone to say something . . ."
2. 12	ERIC	"Yeah, school!"
2. 13	THOMAS	"Something sensible, man."
2. 14	ERIC	"Eh, let's talk about school, man . . ."

2. 15	THOMAS	"School! I been in school four days out of the last two weeks 'cause I got suspended. But . . ."
2. 16	ERIC	"Well that's a . . . You proud a that?"
2. 17	THOMAS	"Nah . . . It's dumb. Why don't we talk about sports then?"
2. 18	WALLACE	"OK!"
2. 19	THOMAS	"These guys wanna talk about football. These guys wanna talk about golf."
2. 20	ERIC	"I don't wanna talk about football."
2. 21	THOMAS	" . . . well then, what do ya' wanna talk about?"
2. 22	ERIC	"Let's talk about something besides sports or video games. Let's talk about something that you would normally talk about in a group."
2. 23	COUNSELOR	"Well, what's important?" QUESTIONING to challenge group thought
2. 24	WALLACE	"Well, there's like ah . . . and"
2. 25	RICK	"Anger management!"
2. 26	WALLACE	"I've had enough of that anger management."
2. 27	COUNSELOR	"Well, what's important? To the people in this group?" QUESTIONING to challenge group thought in context
2. 28	THOMAS	"Money." (Thumb and finger rubbing, money hand gesture.)
2. 29	ERIC	"School, job."
2. 30	COUNSELOR	"Well, a, I hear from some people over here, sports. I hear some people, school, the future." ■ ______________ ● ______________ ▼ ______________
2. 31	THOMAS	"I'm a focused on sports, man. 'cause you know . . . 'cause ah, you gotta be like in shape and everything to be able to play. 'Cause you know my coach made me play."
2. 32	ERIC	"If you think about it . . ."
2. 33	THOMAS	"Thirty-six minutes the last game . . ."
2. 34	ERIC	"Is sports . . ."
2. 35	THOMAS	"Your legs just burn."
2. 36	ERIC	"Is sports a group subject that you usually talk about in a group?"
2. 37	THOMAS	"Yeah, a group of my friends. I don't hafta' go to group. What group I ever been to?"
2. 38	ERIC	"This one. This one right here."

2. 39	THOMAS	"Oh, all right. Well, I know we talk about sports every once in awhile here . . ."
2. 40	COUNSELOR	"Hum. Well, what's it like to be in this group right now?" ■ ______________ ● ______________ ▼ ______________
2. 41	WALLACE	"Weird."
2. 42	THOMAS	"Sorta weird, 'cause nobody got nothin', everything somebody say, nobody else wants to talk about it. Nobody can agree on anything."
2. 43	RICK	"Let's compromise."
2. 44	ERIC	"Usually the counselor will usually have something that we're gonna talk about."
2. 45	RICK	"Let's compromise." *This may be an early example of the group trying to work together.*
2. 46	THOMAS	"Yeah, our mentalities aren't that big, yet, we can't think."
2. 47	COUNSELOR	"So you would feel more comfortable if I took charge of the group right now?" PLAYING A HUNCH to challenge group feeling *In question form*
2. 48	RICK	"Yeah."
2. 49	JAMES	"No. I wouldn't."
2. 50	THOMAS	"I wouldn't 'cause then she'll start talking about stupid stuff, huh?"
2. 51	ERIC	"Why don't we talk about school? Or talk about what's going on at home."
2. 52	RICK	"School? You wanna talk about school? School or grades?"
2. 53	ERIC	"Makes no difference to me."
2. 54	THOMAS	"OK, what's your grades then?"
2. 55	RICK	"Well, let's see, I got a couple of B's, couple of A's and one C."
2. 56	THOMAS	"What grade you in? You only got five periods?"
2. 57	RICK	"No."
2. 58	JAMES	"Are you in special ed.?"
2. 59	RICK	"Three classes." *Note the look on Rick's face.*
2. 60	THOMAS	"You?"
2. 61	JAMES	"One class, but it's easy to get good grades in special ed. 'cause they give you easy work."

2. 62	THOMAS	"Yeah, 'cause I . . ."
2. 63	JAMES	"It doesn't prepare you for your SAT tests because they . . . You going to college? Are you going to college?"
2. 64	RICK	"I don't want to though."
2. 65	WALLACE	"I want to, gotta get an education to get a good job."
2. 66	THOMAS	"I'm going to college, to play basketball, man. I gotta go to college for three years to get drafted, or even signed to get drafted. So, I have to go if I wanna play."
2. 67	THOMAS	"Talk about shoes?"
2. 68	ERIC	"Shoes."
2. 69	THOMAS	"What's the group topic, dude? You don't even know what it is."
2. 70	ERIC	"It's a therapeutic topic, bro. It's a therapeutic deal."
2. 71	THOMAS	"Like get personal."
2. 72	ERIC	"No, don't want to get personal."
2. 73	RICK	"Like at the house or something."
2. 74	ERIC	"Like what happens in your life."
2. 75	COUNSELOR	"What would happen in this group if we talked about something personal?" ■ __________ ● __________ ▼ __________
2. 76	RICK	"Probably be scared." *Note the reflection in Rick's voice of his feeling about what would happen if the group became personal.*
2. 77	THOMAS	"Somebody would start laughing."
2. 78	ERIC	"Ain't nothing gonna happen, ain't nobody gonna start laughing or something. We can all handle it."
2. 79	MITCHELL	"Everybody doesn't wanta hear about everybody's life. I particularly don't want to hear about other people's life."
2. 80	COUNSELOR	"Would you like to tell the group?" QUESTIONING to challenge individual behavior in context
2. 81	ERIC	"Why don't you come up with something, Jennifer? Like I said before, huh?" *Another challenge to the counselor*
2. 82	THOMAS	"She's just sitting here quietly looking around."

2. 83	COUNSELOR	"Yeah, what's that like for you, Thomas, for me to be sitting here quietly?" QUESTIONING to challenge individual experience
2. 84	WALLACE	"We could talk about . . ."
2. 85	THOMAS	"That's the first time I heard my counselor, or any counselor that's around me, be quiet, for real, because they all be on your case."
2. 86	COUNSELOR	"So this is a new experience for you?" PARAPHRASING to acknowledge individual experience *In question form*
2. 87	THOMAS	"Well, no, it doesn't bother me."
2. 88	JAMES	"How long have people been in the system?"
2. 89	RICK	"The YMCA system?"
2. 90	JAMES	"No, the DSHS system."
2. 91	RICK	"DSHS?"
2. 92	ERIC	"The state, man."
2. 93	THOMAS	"I don't know."
2. 94	RICK	"Ever since I was three."
2. 95	ERIC	"How long you been a ward of the state, James?"
2. 96	JAMES	"Since I was three."
2. 97	ERIC	"How bout you?"
2. 98	WALLACE	"Eleven years."
2. 99	ERIC	"How old were you?"
2. 100	THOMAS	"Oh, you talkin about . . ."
2. 101	WALLACE	"Eight years old."
2. 102	THOMAS	". . . I been like nine months. September I moved in . . ."
2. 103	JAMES	"How old are you?"
2. 104	WALLACE	"Fourteen going on 15."
2. 105	THOMAS	"Yeah, September."
2. 106	JAMES	"You think it feels any different than if they had six other kids come in here that weren't in the system? Do you think we'd be talking about other, different, stuff?"
2. 107	RICK	"Yeah."
2. 108	JAMES	"See, I think there's a psychological thing because,"

2. 109	THOMAS	"No, it'd be the same thing."
2. 110	RICK	"No it wouldn't."
2. 111	WALLACE	"Well, it depends."
2. 112	JAMES	"Well, for me there's a psychological difference because I've been in so many group homes and foster homes. Like a couple of years ago I wanted to be able to socialize with my own age group because I wasn't around it, because I was in what I consider captivity in a goddam fucking zoo, OK?"
2. 113	JAMES	"I was locked up . . ."
2. 114	MITCHELL	"I kind of get what he's saying because he's talking about like being like regular kids. If you brought six other regular kids in here, they haven't been, you know . . ."
2. 115	ERIC	"Probably have a brawl going on, man."
2. 116	THOMAS	" . . . for five months."
2. 117	MITCHELL	"They'd be talking about, you know, stuff that goes on."
2. 118	THOMAS	"They'd be talking about the same thing, they'd be talking about sports, school, and home, but the home situation would be different, probably school would be different."
2. 119	ERIC	"Not a hell of a lot different."
2. 120	JAMES	"Yeah, but a whole hell of a lot different because, they probably, they grew up with their parents so their social aspect is different, so they would be talking about different stuff, I know for a fact."
2. 121	COUNSELOR	"So, James, what you are saying is that you feel alike with the other people in group because you feel different." PARAPHRASING to acknowledge individual feeling in context
2. 122	JAMES	"I know for myself that I felt different, then somebody else's different. Different than anybody else because I know, you know, when I go to school I look at other people, and they haven't been in like four group homes and 40 respite, or you know, short term foster placements."
2. 123	THOMAS	"Yeah, duh, I mean like if you look around your school like and you think like, you have a friend, or something, who's like living at home, you know, and obviously it's gonna be different because the situation is different, they learn differently. Like, say they get in trouble and they go home and they get grounded. Say you get in trouble, you go home, and you gotta talk to this dude, this dude. It's a lot different. Your whole life is different. The whole situation is like . . ."
2. 124	WALLACE	"Uh-huh."

2. 125	JAMES	"The thing is, once you learn the system, when you're like in the DSHS system when you get in trouble you just say, you know, 'fuck it, man.'"
2. 126	ERIC	"Personally I think this system sucks."
2. 127	ERIC	"It stinks."
2. 128	COUNSELOR	"Who else in group feels the way that James does?" QUESTIONING to explore group feeling
2. 129	ERIC	"I do."
2. 130	THOMAS	"I don't think it's worth it though, 'cause you know . . ."
2. 131	ERIC	"Other people, you can't really define normal, but half the time I don't feel normal, 'cause you can't. I mean, being in the system you don't got as many opportunities as most other kids do."
2. 132	THOMAS	"Well I think actually you do."
2. 133	JAMES	"You ain't got that family set either because you don't have a dad, like most of the time you don't have a brother or a sister, and so, a grandma or grandpa . . ."
2. 134	ERIC	"A normal person should be able to count on . . ."
2. 135	JAMES	"You don't sociologically, you know, develop man. You don't, you can't picture that, so it's hard for you to fit into a setting, mold in it, especially when you're like 15, 16 years old."
2. 136	ERIC	"But a normal person should be able to always count, always count on two people in their life, their mom and their dad, to always love them, to always be there."
2. 137	RICK	"I got two moms."
2. 138	THOMAS	"Oh, stepmom and real mom?"
2. 139	WALLACE	"No, two moms in one house."
2. 140	RICK	"Two moms."
2. 141	ERIC	"Two moms? How can anyone have two moms?"
2. 142	RICK	"As in a lesbian relationship, gay lesbian relationship, committed to each other . . ."
2. 143	ERIC	"How did we jump from talking about . . ."
2. 144	JAMES	"Yo, who's this 'we' brother, what are you talking about?"
2. 145	RICK	"Oh, I live with two moms."
2. 146	JAMES	"That must be . . ."
2. 147	ERIC	"They lesbians?"

2. 148	MITCHELL	"Yeah, they are but . . ."
2. 149	WALLACE	"Yeah, and you know, they're actually quite normal."
2. 150	RICK	"They are, they . . ."
2. 151	ERIC	"Is it, different?"
2. 152	WALLACE	"No."
2. 153	MITCHELL	"They're two females but I think for these two guys they have more affection in the house 'cause there's two women . . ." *Note their discussion about how they perceive the foster mothers.*
2. 154	ERIC	"Well, in foster care it's harder to find someone that you can always count on."
2. 155	THOMAS	"I think you're more independent, dude, 'cause, you know, you got a lot more you gotta handle on your own now."
2. 156	ERIC	"That too."
2. 157	THOMAS	"Especially at home. 'Cause you know at home your parents take more care of you because, for one thing, they're, they're, they've known you for so long. And they've been raising you . . ."
2. 158	ERIC	"Well, like kids that aren't in the system, just for an example, stuff like getting your license and a car, and taking driver's ed."
2. 159	WALLACE	"You usually get your driver's permit . . ."
2. 160	ERIC	"Usually normal parents, they'll like help pay for it or pay all of it for their kid and, I mean, a foster kid's gotta pay for all of it themselves."
2. 161	ERIC	"You can't count on, there's nobody to count on for stuff like that."
2. 162	WALLACE	" . . . and usually half the time with the program you don't get your driver's license until you're 18."
2. 163	WALLACE	"Which really sucks."
2. 164	THOMAS	"I'm getting my . . ."
2. 165	ERIC	"That's one reason I don't feel normal."
2. 166	THOMAS	"I'm getting my driver's license . . ."
2. 167	COUNSELOR	"What about counting on people . . . in the group?" QUESTIONING to challenge individual behavior in context
2. 168	THOMAS	"Huh? Counting on people in the group?"
2. 169	COUNSELOR	"Can't you count on people in this group, right now?" ■ ________ ● ________ ▼ ________
2. 170	JAMES	"You changed the subject." *Note James' awareness of the change in the group.*

2. 171	JAMES	"Keep on talking, what are you all talking about?"
2. 172	THOMAS	"It's like this. If you have, like, a bunch of friends, right? And say like, a, the other day on the bus, . . . I forgot, I have to carry a progress report because in case you get in trouble your parents gotta know about it. Ah, I forgot to get it signed, like all day."
2. 173	ERIC	"See there's another thing that make you feel unnormal."
2. 174	THOMAS	"Yeah, well."
2. 175	ERIC	"Have your teacher sign the damn thing."
2. 176	THOMAS	"Yeah. Hey, can you please sign this? I'm a bad kid . . ."
2. 177	WALLACE	"Especially when they say it out loud, it's like what's this for."
2. 178	THOMAS	"My parents need to know what I'm doing all the time."
2. 179	ERIC	"That's like, that's, if you've gotta bring a progress report to school all the time, that's just gonna make your foster parents or somebody think, or your teachers think that you're bad."
2. 180	THOMAS	"Unless you can afford to do well."
2. 181	ERIC	"Well, why would he have to bring a progress report to school if he ain't bad?"
2. 182	JAMES	"I got something here. Another thing."
2. 183	JAMES	"When I play football, when I go on that field, I'm bringing more intensity and more."
2. 184	ERIC	"See, you're jumping back to sports, right?"
2. 185	THOMAS	"He's back into sports."
2. 186	JAMES	"I've never had any parents, OK, so those other kids go out there. I don't know what the hell they're trying to do. I'm going out there, focus on one thing, and that's to do the best of my ability that I can."
2. 187	ERIC	"Now you're talking about sports again."
2. 188	JAMES	"Since, because you know, it just like, I think for that it gives me an advantage in football. I don't know, I'm just saying this because, you know, I got no parents."
2. 189	ERIC	"OK, what you're trying to say is not having stuff makes you a stronger person, and it does."
2. 190	MITCHELL	"It does."
2. 191	ERIC	"Makes you stronger mentally."
2. 192	JAMES	"But then I go out on the football field . . . And another thing is though is since, you know, is since, and another thing that pisses

		me off is since I've never had any parents, I try to prove to people, like my coach, like when I was at Cascade High School. I liked him 'cause he said, he'd come up to me in the hall, 'How's it going, James?' and all of this. And that give me a pat on the back, you know, and, you know I look up to people like that."
2. 193	THOMAS	"Oh, I get it. Like teachers who are against you like find out about your situation and then, like, no leeway at all. They found out about my situation, he used to like, give me slack and everything, then it was like referral, referral, referral, you know, he was like, and he like talks in front of the class 'I'm gonna call your foster parents, or somethin.' Then my teacher said, 'I'm gonna call the yunnie,' and I was like 'What?' And all the kids start ranking on you and they bug you and, you know, it's like lots of peer pressure 'cause the teacher's got a big ole mouth."
2. 194	ERIC	"That's one thing I don't like. Like people, like a lot of kids I know that are in the system, they've got friends at school but most of their friends, they don't know they're in a foster home, they don't know they got foster parents."
2. 195	MITCHELL	"'cause that's not, personally, I don't think that's none of their business."
2. 196	ERIC	"Yeah, but why would you lie to your friends?"
2. 197	THOMAS	"It's not cool."
2. 198	ERIC	"But, listen, if you lie to your friends about something like that . . ."
2. 199	THOMAS	"They find out."
2. 200	ERIC	"No, not that they find out, but you don't know that they're your real friends 'cause they don't know you for who you are. How do you know they like you for who you are?"
2. 201	MITCHELL	"My friends now know who I am and still . . ."
2. 202	THOMAS	"How many friends do you have?"
2. 203	MITCHELL	"Me? I have a lot of friends for coming to a new school. I got a lot of friends quick, 'cause I make friends easily, but still people going around running their mouths about this and that saying . . . running their . . . when I could tell them, that doesn't help out at all. If you take time you wanna learn who you're trusting, 'cause if you don't tell them right away, that gives you time to learn the person, you know what they're like, you know, if you see somebody?"
2. 204	ERIC	"I've told every single friend I have at school."
2. 205	THOMAS	"Ah man, I've had like four girls chase me down yesterday."
2. 206	ERIC	" . . . everybody, and they don't care."

2. 207	THOMAS	"'cause I was so good at basketball."
2. 208	ERIC	"If you're gonna have friends that like you for who you are, not for what you have, or . . ."
2. 209	MITCHELL	"People have acquaintances, people that they just talk to, not all your business, and that. If you don't wanna tell them, then other people shouldn't either."
2. 210	ERIC	"The really popular kids at school are either athletes, they get recognized for their athletic skills, or . . ."
2. 211	THOMAS	"Everybody talks to me . . ."
2. 212	ERIC	"Or singing in talent shows or break dancing, whatever. Everybody, they start liking them 'cause they're good at something."
2. 213	JAMES	"That's what I'm talking about . . . When I didn't have parent figures, that's why, what I'm talking about, when I go on the football field that's what I'm trying to do. I'm trying to get people to recognize me, especially like the coaches, you know?"
2. 214	JAMES	"Like my foster dad, I don't consider him a father figure, OK, because half the time the motherfucker can't even hear me. I tell him to fuck off, he's in his fucking room and like hey man, ignores me and walks into his fucking room . . ."
2. 215	ERIC	"He's not trying to take the place of your dad, guy, he's not a father figure."
2. 216	JAMES	"That's why when I go to school, man, when I play sports, that's why I try to do my best, you know, and sometimes I get mad, you know, and like that, and I go crazy and the people are just like, oh man . . ."
2. 217	THOMAS	"Like a real parent would back you up and everything and like at a sports game, you know, be all cheering for you. Your foster parent sitting up there smoking a cigarette or something, off to the side."
2. 218	JAMES	"Or at home sleeping."
2. 219	MITCHELL	". . . the only thing, the only thing."
2. 220	THOMAS	"And he don't give me a key to the house so he want me to stay outside, so I went to my friend's . . ."
2. 221	ERIC	"That's what I'm saying, man, I got, you know I went to jail 'cause I climbed in my bedroom window 'cause he wasn't home."
2. 222	THOMAS	"Oh my god. After the police . . ."
2. 223	COUNSELOR	"There's a real theme in this group about not feeling important." ■ ______________ ● ______________ ▼ ______________
2. 224	THOMAS	"Well, I feel important."

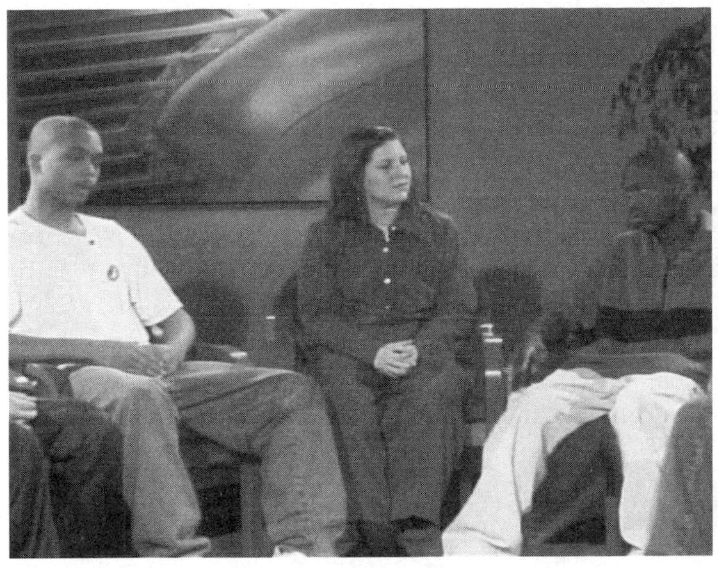

2. 225	RICK	"I don't feel important."
2. 226	ERIC	"You don't feel like you got anybody there, like family, or . . ."
2. 227	THOMAS	"Real close, somebody . . . you can talk to . . ."
2. 228	ERIC	"You know, nobody close that you can relate to, talk to."
2. 229	THOMAS	"Like my grandma, I can talk to her."
2. 230	ERIC	"That will be always be there and you know that no matter what will always be there and care about you. Most kids in foster homes don't have that."
2. 231	JAMES	"That's another thing, man, when I go into the weight room I get so mad and I go in there and I see, no,"
2. 232	ERIC	"Talking about sports and shit . . ."
2. 233	JAMES	"Yeah, but still this,"
2. 234	MITCHELL	"He's talking about his life . . ."
2. 235	JAMES	"That's the only thing, though, is when I walk in there I see all these other kids, they got a mom and a dad and they go in there and I don't even know what they're trying to lift the weights for because when I go in there, man, I'm trying to prove, you know, to everybody in that whole weight room, which I don't think those other kids are . . . that."
2. 236	THOMAS	"That you're cool."
2. 237	JAMES	"No, I'm trying to be strong, you know, and I just go in there to try to get people to recognize who I am."

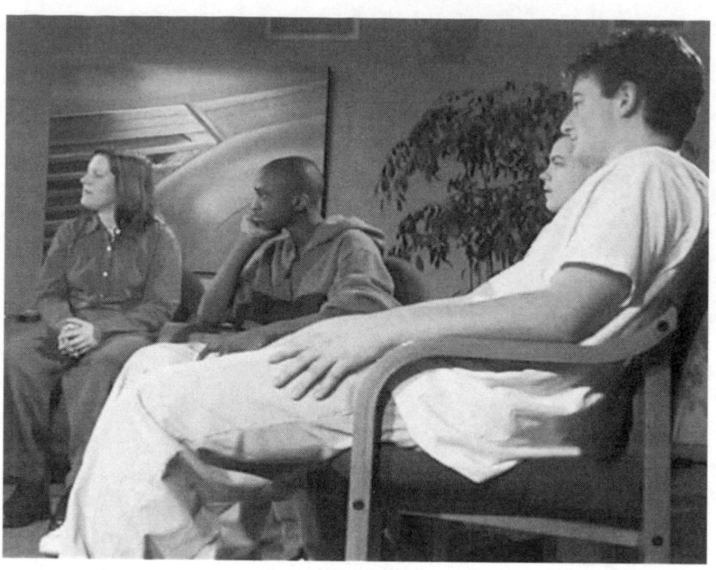

2. 238	COUNSELOR	"I'd like to stop the group and go back to what Rick was saying." DIRECTING to challenge group behavior
2. 239	RICK	"I was referring to you, when I was trying to say something, but I got interrupted, but that's OK. I was trying to say that so you mean that you go into the gym to work out your anger and also prove that you're someone?"
2. 240	JAMES	(nodding) "Um-hmm."
2. 241	WALLACE	"I do that every time . . ."
2. 242	JAMES	"Which I feel when I go in there that no one else is bringing that in there."
2. 243	ERIC	"So you wanna feel important?"
2. 244	THOMAS	"You wanna look bad."
2. 245	JAMES	"I wanna look bad."
2. 246	ERIC	"You wanna be somebody."
2. 247	JAMES	"I wanna be somebody."
2. 248	COUNSELOR	"How can you . . . ?" *An interrupted counselor response*
2. 249	JAMES	"But those other people just go out there, I don't know what they're going out there for, just, you know, just to be good . . ."
2. 250	ERIC	"Most people will go into a weight room to lift weights, you know, and build their body."
2. 251	THOMAS	"Most people don't have to worry about looking good."

2. 252	COUNSELOR	"There's, well there's no weights in group though, so how can you be strong in group? There's no weights, there's no exercise room here." QUESTIONING to challenge individual behavior in context
2. 253	ERIC	"You've gotta be mentally strong."
2. 254	WALLACE	"Yeah."
2. 255	MITCHELL	"You've gotta have positive feedback."
2. 256	THOMAS	"And you gotta be able to take in what people throw at you and put it back out, you know? Like somebody, say, give their opinion about you and you gotta be able to take that in."
2. 257	MITCHELL	"If somebody says something in group . . ."
2. 258	WALLACE	"Or just say something mean back to them."
2. 259	MITCHELL	"You should say, you know, you shouldn't say something mean back to them. You should say something positive. Maybe they're feeling down or something about something and if you throw something positive back at 'em then it might change their train of thought."
2. 260	RICK	"If someone's feeling bad you can also comfort them by saying that you know how they feel, but like you've been in the same situation."
2. 261	THOMAS	"That's more like a . . ."
2. 262	MITCHELL	"Was everybody not here in this room put in this world by themselves? So you should rely on yourself. If you rely on other people . . ."
2. 263	ERIC	"You're not put in this world by yourself, man."
2. 264	MITCHELL	"Hey, did you come out with smarts? Did you come out with genius?"
2. 265	THOMAS	"Somebody teach you."
2. 266	MITCHELL	"Did you come out with a IQ?"
2. 267	ERIC	"It's called genetics, bro."
2. 268	MITCHELL	"When you go through life, are you always going to expect for your parents to be there for you?"
2. 269	ERIC	"No."
2. 270	MITCHELL	"Or anybody else?"
2. 271	ERIC	"You shouldn't expect it, but most kids do."
2. 272	MITCHELL	"OK, especially for, OK, you guys were in the system since you were three, right?"

2. 273	ERIC	"I've been in the system for 14 years."
2. 274	MITCHELL	"OK, so how old were you?"
2. 275	MITCHELL	"So all three of you guys, were you in here for a long time too?"
2. 276	WALLACE	"I've been in here for like, 10, 11, 12 years."
2. 277	COUNSELOR	"I notice there's a lot of giggling when we're talking about serious stuff like how long we've been in the system." GIVING FEEDBACK to acknowledge group behavior *While this is the response of GIVING FEEDBACK, it does point out a possible discrepancy.*
2. 278	MITCHELL	"Hey look, you three . . ."
2. 279	COUNSELOR	"Maybe not giggling, snickering." *Not a counseling response*
2. 280	MITCHELL	"You three out of all people you say you don't care about your mom, right?"
2. 281	ERIC	"Me?"
2. 282	MITCHELL	"Yeah."
2. 283	ERIC	"I don't know my mom."
2. 284	MITCHELL	"See, do you know your parents?"
2. 285	WALLACE	"I don't care about my dad."
2. 286	MITCHELL	"Do you know your parents?"
2. 287	THOMAS	"Most people."
2. 288	MITCHELL	"Look, you guys, especially you guys, three, should be real strong and have that thought where you were put, 'cause for all three of you guys you were put here by yourself, meaning that you don't know your mom, or anybody . . ."
2. 289	WALLACE	"I know my mom."
2. 290	MITCHELL	"I mean all you have is DSHS."
2. 291	COUNSELOR	"Mitchell, is that how you feel?" QUESTIONING to challenge individual feeling
2. 292	ERIC	"You weren't brought into the world by yourself, you didn't bring yourself into this world, you know."
2. 293	THOMAS	"No, no, no, I think what he's trying to say is nobody was there to help him, like . . ."
2. 294a	COUNSELOR	"I'm gonna stop you all for a second. Mitchell. Excuse me. Mitchell, is that how you feel?"

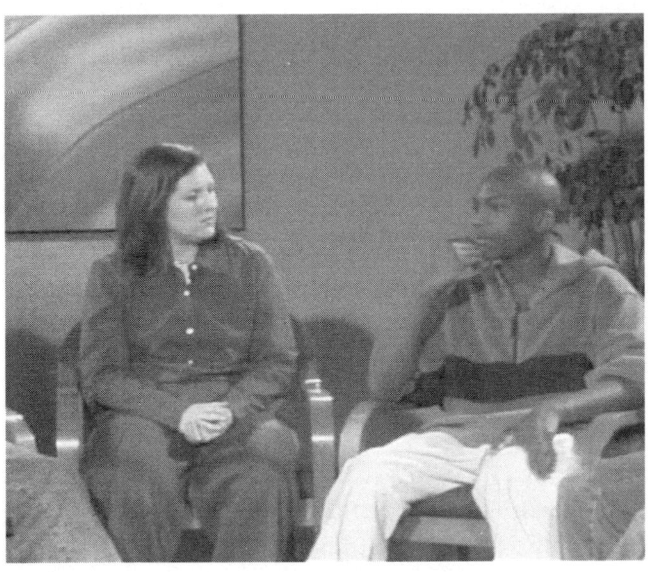

2. 294b		DIRECTING to challenge group behavior QUESTIONING to challenge individual feeling *Note the combination of responses.*
2. 295	MITCHELL	"No, I'm saying . . ."
2. 296	COUNSELOR	"How do you feel for yourself?" QUESTIONING to challenge individual feeling
2. 297	MITCHELL	"For me, I have people, you know. Sometimes I don't use that to my, to my, you know, whatever I need, but I have people to talk to, like role models, family, people. But I mean for people that don't, they should think about, you know, trying to stick up for themselves. Like James, he's sitting here saying that he's sports, and you're saying that you know, whatever, or whatever, but he's sitting here saying that he's put here, you know, and he's trying to make a role for himself, you know, and then his future he can have something for his kids, you know, and so they're gonna have something."
2. 298	COUNSELOR	"So how do you feel about what he said?" ■ ______________ ● ______________ ▼ ______________
2. 299 ⬇	MITCHELL	"I'm like taking that in, and that like, I think of him as a better person now 'cause he's talking about that. I mean he's like, he's sittin' here saying he doesn't know, he knows us three, and maybe him, you know, but he's sitting here saying exactly how he feels, whatever, and other people are, like, like backing up and he's just letting it out. He's saying exactly, you know, he's not cuttin' any bull, he's getting straight to the point."

2. 300a 2. 300b	COUNSELOR	"So you respect him being real in group. And what about the rest of the group?" PARAPHRASE to acknowledge individual thought in context QUESTIONING to challenge group thought
2. 301	WALLACE	"I was trying to say something, but I got cut off . . ."
2. 302	ERIC	"I'm being real."
2. 303	WALLACE	"You know like how he said that people liked him because he played basketball?"
2. 304	COUNSELOR	"Tell the whole group, Wallace." DIRECTING to challenge individual behavior
2. 305	WALLACE	" . . . Well, you see, one time I went out to try to play soccer. Nobody liked me until they figured out how hard I could kick a soccer ball. Everybody started hanging out with me, just 'cause I could kick a soccer ball really hard, kick a football really hard."
2. 306	THOMAS	"People used to hang out with me 'cause I was tall."
2. 307	COUNSELOR	"So you were really sympathizing with what he was saying?" EMPATHIZING to acknowledge individual feeling *In question form*
2. 308	WALLACE	"Yeah, and like one time I was playing football and the dude passed me and I like ran fast and nobody could catch me so everybody wanted me on their team 'cause I was fast."
2. 309	THOMAS	"Yeah, sorta like . . ."
2. 310	MITCHELL	"Not 'cause they knew you . . ."
2. 311	WALLACE	"Yeah, that's what I'm saying."
2. 312	COUNSELOR	"Well, I'm hearing a lot about how people feel that they can have status and be confident outside of group, but I've only heard one person, Mitchell, say that to be real in group is something to respect right now." GIVING FEEDBACK to acknowledge group behavior with immediacy in context
2. 313	THOMAS	"Yeah, what I think he's trying to say is . . ."
2. 314	ERIC	"It's not easy to come out here and talk about your life and talk about how you feel. You don't know if somebody's gonna laugh . . ."
2. 315	WALLACE	"I mean it's not that easy. Most people don't wanna talk about their family issues."
2. 316	JAMES	"I'm trying to relate to that."
2. 317	JAMES	"Like Randy Moss. He came from a single mother."

2. 318	THOMAS	"Who?"
2. 319	JAMES	"And, you know, he, you know, he had a hard life, he had a kid when he was in his teens."
2. 320	THOMAS	"Ohhhh."
2. 321	JAMES	"He did some drugs. He went to college, he's, I don't know if somebody broke that national record, but he set some national records for college division one. Came out of Marshall University. People passed him up in the draft."
2. 322	COUNSELOR	"Excuse me." DIRECTING to challenge individual behavior
2. 323	JAMES	"No, in the draft . . ."
2. 324	COUNSELOR	"Excuse me, James." DIRECTING to challenge individual behavior
2. 325	JAMES	"In the draft . . ."
2. 326	COUNSELOR	"Excuse me, James." DIRECTING to challenge individual behavior
2. 327	JAMES	"Because of his background, because . . ."
2. 328	ERIC	"James, James!"
2. 329	JAMES	"So then the Minnesota Vikings picked him up . . ."
2. 330	COUNSELOR	"So, James, how do you feel about me interrupting you right now." QUESTIONING to challenge individual feeling with immediacy
2. 331	JAMES	"I can relate to that . . ."
2. 332	COUNSELOR	"James?"
2. 333	JAMES	"See that's what I'm trying to show, you know."
2. 334	COUNSELOR	"James, how do you feel about me interrupting you right now?" ■ ______________ ● ______________ ▼ ______________
2. 335	JAMES	"Well, what are you interrupting me for? Go ahead, go ahead."
2. 336	MITCHELL	"Because we were just trying to say in the draft, in the draft."
2. 337	COUNSELOR	"You just wanted to say that? But before you were talking about how that applied to you and how that applied to about the way you feel, and now you're talking about . . ." PARAPHRASING to explore individual behavior
2. 338	JAMES	"But you know why that happened is because you jumped in before when he was gonna say something."

2. 339	COUNSELOR	"Uh-huh." ATTENDING to acknowledge individual experience
2.340	JAMES	"And then you jumped in after that and you changed the whole discussion around."
2. 341	THOMAS	"How do you feel about her jumping in front of you like that?" *Note the counseling response.*
2. 342	JAMES	"I don't have a problem, but I don't see what you're . . ."
2. 343	THOMAS	"Does it irritate you or what? I think what everybody's trying to say . . ."
2. 344	COUNSELOR	"How about the group? How does the group feel about what happened between James and I?" ■ ______________ ● ______________ ▼ ______________
2. 345	THOMAS	"I think that James was trying to make a point and it's hard to talk in this group because everybody's talkin', so he wanted to get it in before he was done talking, because if you would have interrupted him . . ." *Note Thomas' paraphrase of what has happened. This may be a real therapeutic moment since his behavior starts to change in the group at this point.*
2. 346	COUNSELOR	"But how did you feel, Thomas, when I interrupted James?" QUESTIONING to challenge individual feeling in context
2. 347	THOMAS	"Well,"
2. 348	COUNSELOR	"How do you feel right now?" QUESTIONING to challenge individual feeling with immediacy
2. 349	THOMAS	"I feel fine, why? How 'm I 'spose to feel? If you were to interrupt me like that, I wouldn't like it because . . ."
2. 350	COUNSELOR	"You wouldn't like it?" EMPATHIZING to acknowledge individual feeling
2. 351	THOMAS	"I'd want a reason why you're interrupting me. But, you know, I'd been waiting to talk and you know, it would sort of irritate me, but I'd probably be quiet."
2. 352	COUNSELOR	"So, you would feel irritated, but you wouldn't show it to me that you were irritated?" PARAPHRASING to acknowledge individual feeling and behavior
2. 353	THOMAS	"I would show it to you after you interrupted me, started hitting on me, but otherwise, no way."
2. 354	COUNSELOR	"OK, Eric." *Not a counseling response*

2. 355	ERIC	"Now I forgot what I was gonna say. Oh, I think you had a good reason for interrupting James because he was going on about irrelevant about what we're talking about."
2. 356	JAMES	"But it wasn't irrelevant . . ."
2. 357	THOMAS	"I don't agree it's irrelevant."
2. 358	ERIC	"You were talking about a sports hero . . ."
2. 359	JAMES	"But he's not a hero . . ."
2. 360	ERIC	"And you're not saying anything about yourself." *This is an example of a group member GIVING FEEDBACK that may be challenging.*
2. 361	JAMES	"Look at his background, look at his background, look where he came from."
2. 362	MITCHELL	"He is, he said he was his role model."
2. 363	ERIC	"Makes no difference."
2. 364	JAMES	"He came from like a single mother family."
2. 365	ERIC	"You're not relating that to you . . ."
2. 366	JAMES	"He came from the ghetto and look where he is and people would pass him up because, you know . . ."
2. 367	ERIC	"I think you're not relating . . ."
2. 368	MITCHELL	"He did earlier though, he said that . . ."
2. 369	COUNSELOR	"Eric, so how did you feel when I interrupted him?" QUESTIONING to challenge individual feeling in context
2. 370	ERIC	"When you interrupted?"
2. 371	COUNSELOR	"Uh-huh. How do you feel right now?" QUESTIONING to challenge individual feeling with immediacy
2. 372	THOMAS	"Fine."
2. 373	ERIC	"Fine."
2. 374	COUNSELOR	"You say fine, and then you laugh, so I'm not sure what that means." NOTING A DISCREPANCY to challenge individual behavior
2. 375	THOMAS	"It's like sort of a weird question because you weren't directing it towards us."
2. 376	ERIC	"That question is weird, like how do you feel right now. It's a weird question. I feel fine."

2. 377	COUNSELOR	"So, it's weird because?" QUESTIONING to explore individual thought
2. 378	ERIC	"Because? You mean?"
2. 379	THOMAS	"Because he didn't get interrupted, you interrupted him."
2. 380	ERIC	"Well, because if someone asks how you feel, that's just weird. I don't know why."
2. 381	JAMES	"OK, let me bring up something."
2. 382	COUNSELOR	"So . . . " *Incomplete counselor response*
2. 383	ERIC	"It's not like if you're mad or sad you can just oh I'm mad or I'm sad, but I feel fine."
2. 384	COUNSELOR	"So, you felt uncomfortable 'cause you weren't sure what I wanted you to say?" EMPATHIZING to acknowledge individual feeling
2. 385	ERIC	"No."
2. 386	COUNSELOR	"No?"
2. 387	ERIC	"I feel fine."
2. 388	COUNSELOR	"You feel fine?" EMPATHIZING to acknowledge individual feeling *In question form*
2. 389	MITCHELL	"Counselor, can I say something now?"
2. 390	COUNSELOR	"Please do." *Not a counseling response*
2. 391	MITCHELL	"On that point, Eric, James was sitting here saying that Randy Moss it is, and he might have gone off a little bit, but he was going back to where he was saying that, he does, you know he runs and stuff? Randy Moss is like his role model and he takes Randy Moss, some of his stuff and puts it into his . . ."
2. 392	ERIC	"But he never said that."
2. 393	MITCHELL	"'Cause he hadn't gone there, 'cause he had gone off a little bit, and he was starting to come back."
2. 394	COUNSELOR	"But Mitchell, how did you feel when I interrupted James?" QUESTIONING to challenge individual feeling in context
2. 395	MITCHELL	"I mean that was, I mean, he was kind of rude for him to keep saying stuff but . . ."
2. 396	THOMAS	"How did you feel when he interrupt ya, let's see how did I feel?"

2. 397	JAMES	"OK, let me spit something out, let me spit something out because I . . ."
2. 398	COUNSELOR	"I'm not hearing from the whole group." GIVING FEEDBACK to acknowledge subgroup behavior
2. 399	JAMES	"I don't know where you're trying to come from, Counselor, but were you guys all placed in the DSHS system because of abuse or were you in there for abuse?"
2. 400	JAMES	"Were you in there for abuse?"
2. 401	THOMAS	"What are you talking about, CPS?"
2. 402	JAMES	"Were you tooken away from your parents for any reason?"
2. 403	ERIC	"Why, why aren't you with your parents now?"
2. 404	THOMAS	"Oh, 'cause I got in trouble."
2. 405	ERIC	"So you're not like . . ."
2. 406	JAMES	"How old were you when you were taken away from your parents?"
2. 407	THOMAS	"Well, I wasn't taken away. I got put in a group home 'cause my parents felt like they they couldn't, they felt like I wasn't really, a, really working at home, yeah, stable at home."
2. 408	JAMES	"Mitchell?"
2. 409	MITCHELL	"Same thing as him."
2. 410	JAMES	"Were you taken away from your parents when you were little?"
2. 411	WALLACE	"Yeah."
2. 412	JAMES	"You two are different because I don't know about that because right here, I was taken away from my parents for abuse."
2. 413	WALLACE	"Same here."
2. 414	JAMES	"When I was three years old."
2. 415	THOMAS	"Oh, yeah, CPS? They were at my house a lot."
2. 416	JAMES	"And when you're three years old that's when you're learning, you know, you kind of know how to walk, and you're learning how to talk, so that's like a maturity from like age three to five is a big learning level, right there."
2. 417	THOMAS	"You're not in school."
2. 418	JAMES	"And then, see, they took me away from my parents and put me in this, a, they were going to adopt me and I lived there until I was nine years old. And since that step from age three to five, you know, because I was abused until I was three years old, and so from three to nine years old I still kind of, you know, kind of had that in my

		head when I got abused. I'd be rebelling, I would get an attitude, I wouldn't follow what people said because of what happened to me in my life. Now what they did is they took me out of that and they put me into a group home with other people that had problems because of something like that and I was nine years old and put a nine-year-old with a bunch of 12-year-olds, that are, you know, ruthless and a bunch of criminals beating the shit out of each other, and jostling each other, that's gonna psychologically, you know . . ."
2. 419	THOMAS	"Mess you up?"
2. 420	JAMES	"Mold that into your brain, so it's hard to get that up. So where I am right now is I was tooken away."
2. 421	RICK	"Why are you looking at me?"
2. 422	JAMES	"No."
2. 423	JAMES	I'm just, you know, I can't look like this. I try to do the whole group, but see, they put me in group homes and then they try to say 'James, you know, you gotta problem. We're gonna work on it.' I ain't got a problem, it's just that you took me out of a bad environment and tried to stick me into another one with people that didn't know what they were doing and then you stick me into a group home with other kids that have bad problems and I'm nine years old."
2. 424	COUNSELOR	"So, James, let's speed up for a second to today, right now." DIRECTING to challenge individual behavior with immediacy
2. 425	JAMES	"So, no, so how did you guys revolve around that? About what you said?"
2. 426	COUNSELOR	"So, so how do you, I'm asking you, how do you feel telling the whole group about yourself?" QUESTIONING to challenge individual feeling in context
2. 427	JAMES	"It's not a problem, it's just, you know it's one of those things that makes me mad is because like 'James, you know, you gotta problem we're gonna work on it' and it makes me feel like, you know, that you know I got sent to group home is all's out there smokin' marijuana, you know, or jack somebody's car."
2. 428	COUNSELOR	"So, are you wondering if they feel the same way that you do, right now in group?" QUESTIONING to challenge individual feeling in context with immediacy
2. 429	JAMES	"Yeah, I'm trying to figure out if they kinda feel like that."
2. 430	WALLACE	"Not really, 'cause . . ."
2. 431	JAMES	". . . these guys"
2. 432	WALLACE	"I don't."

2. 433	THOMAS	"I understand what you're saying because, I think what he's trying to say is like, he's sayin when you're born, a, people talkin' to the baby can like help it out, influence it, it's all influence and everything was like when he was young he had bad influence. You know, people, when you're born, you don't know anything, right, you're just kinda googoo, right . . ."
2. 434	THOMAS	"Then people slowly tell you how to talk and influence you, but when you're getting beat on, all you think about is getting beat, you know. Or beating somebody."
2. 435	COUNSELOR	"Thomas can you relate to James when he was telling that story?" QUESTIONING to explore individual feeling
2. 436	THOMAS	"Yeah, sort of because my dad, like when I was young, like three, four, no two, three, and four, he was a pretty violent guy when he got mad, so, a, you know, it sorta influenced me, you know, like that when like I got taken out of that situation, and I knew that I had some freedom, that I wouldn't let nobody do it again, so I like rebelled somebody tried to do something like and like go off real quick, you know? Like have a short temper and everything."
2. 437	COUNSELOR	"Uh-huh." ATTENDING to acknowledge group experience
2. 438	THOMAS	"'Cause like when I got put in a group home, I moved from one situation to another and in this situation there was, you know, you feel more like you have to do what your parents say, but when you're not with your parents and you're with some other adults, it's more easy for you to show what you're really feelin'."
2. 439	COUNSELOR	"So, what's it like to tell the group about that right now?" QUESTIONING to challenge individual feeling in context with immediacy
2. 440	THOMAS	"Well, I think the reason's pretty easy to tell everybody that is because we all are here, we all are in the same program because we've all had some kind of problem, so there's nobody who could be proud, like if he says his problem like this, there's nobody sittin' in here that could say 'well, ha ha' or laugh at him, because they've had something like that happen to them. So,"
2. 441	ERIC	"We can all relate 'cause we're all pretty much in the same . . ."
2. 442	THOMAS	"Even if it's a different problem."
2. 443	WALLACE	"Yeah, I hear."
2. 444	THOMAS	"It's still sorta related."
2. 445	COUNSELOR	"So, but Mitchell's sitting over here saying he's not relating." ■ __________ ● __________ ▼ __________

2. 446	MITCHELL	"I haven't been abused or hit. I mean, if I could, I can't understand, to what?"
2. 447	THOMAS	"Influence, have you when you were growing up."
2. 448	MITCHELL	"I was influenced . . ."
2. 449	THOMAS	"Did people do things in front of you, like smoke or something?"
2. 450	MITCHELL	"When I was younger, my mom, I grew up in real holy house, you know. So, like everything that I saw was revolved around God and just it was you know . . ."
2. 451	THOMAS	"What're you doin' here?"
2. 452	MITCHELL	"If you're bad . . ."
2. 453	ERIC	"What I mean, like, oh I interrupt, but what I mean is like now we're all in a foster home."
2. 454	WALLACE	"Right."
2. 455	MITCHELL	"I can relate with the foster home, not the same reason we're all here, but I can relate that we're all in a foster home."
2. 456	THOMAS	"I just don't understand, I just don't understand that why, he's I don't understand why . . ."
2. 457	MITCHELL	"It seems like . . ."
2. 458	JAMES	"No he's gonna go next."
2. 459	ERIC	"We went from how we felt about saying this stuff . . ."
2. 460	WALLACE	"I wanna speak too." *Interrupted response*
2. 461	COUNSELOR	"You notice the group did a . . ."
2. 462	JAMES	"No, no, what happened is I said what I said and he said that he couldn't relate to it because he wasn't in that environment . . ."
2. 463	COUNSELOR	"Well, I'm gonna stop you . . ." DIRECTING to challenge individual behavior
2. 464	JAMES	". . . see that's OK"
2. 465	COUNSELOR	"Excuse me James. I'm gonna stop you. Could you say more about that, Eric?" DIRECTING to challenge individual behavior
2. 466	ERIC	"Well we were all talkin' about, or you were asking how he felt about talkin' about, you know, your life and your childhood and how you feel about that, and you were askin' how you feel about sayin' that to a group."

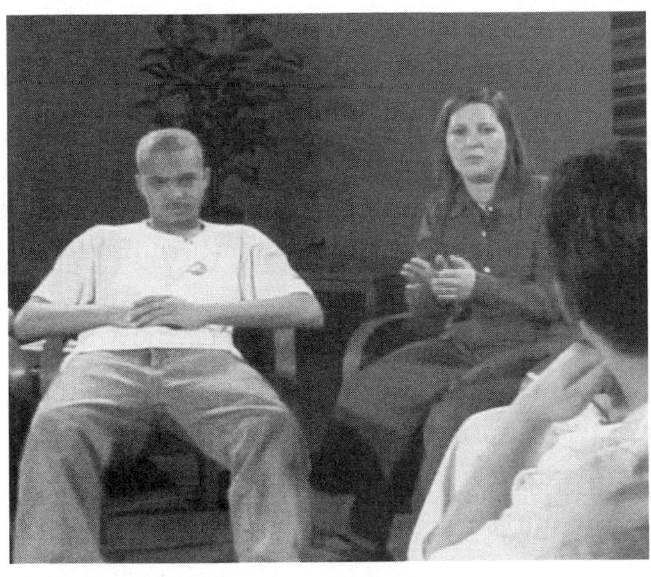

2. 467	COUNSELOR	"Yes." *Not a counseling response*
2. 468	ERIC	"And then it just all kinda jumped off and got in this whole argument/conversation thing over it."
2. 469	JAMES	"No, because what happened is what I said, in, I kinda wasn't kinda talkin' to you too because . . ."
2. 470	COUNSELOR	"James, could you respond to what Eric's saying? He's saying that . . ." DIRECTING to challenge individual behavior
2. 471	ERIC	"She asked the question."
2. 472	JAMES	"Yeah, because what happened is now, what I said, it was meant for you, you and him, because you guys kinda really were in that environment, so then Mitchell said he couldn't relate to that because his mom was a . . ."
2. 473	COUNSELOR	"James, do you notice that you're still doing what Eric pointed out a minute ago, that we were talking about what it felt like to talk about this in group and that people went and started talking about other things, not about feelings. And you're still talking about the facts of the conversation. Not the feeling, but what it's like to be in this group." NOTING A CONNECTION to challenge individual behavior in context
2. 474	JAMES	"Oh, I'm talking about the feeling, he's feeling . . ."
2. 475	COUNSELOR	"OK, well maybe I'm missing that. I'm asking how you're feeling about being." QUESTIONING to challenge individual feeling

2. 476	JAMES	"How I'm feeling?"
2. 477	COUNSELOR	"Yes." *Not a counseling response*
2. 478	JAMES	"Oh, I'm feelin', I'm feelin' just fine, you know."
2. 479	ERIC	"She was askin' how it feels to talk about your past and stuff in this group."
2. 480	JAMES	"Oh, it's not a problem, you know."
2. 481	COUNSELOR	"So you feel very comfortable saying this . . ." EMPATHIZING to acknowledge individual feeling
2. 482	JAMES	"Oh, I feel very comfortable, what I'm just tryin' to do is for to you to be quiet for a second because I . . . no don't say anything because . . ."
2. 483	ERIC	"You're getting off the subject."
2. 484	JAMES	"Well, he was talking. Were you not relating, saying you couldn't relate to what I kinda said?"
2. 485	MITCHELL	"Yeah, and then he mentioned that well, why can't you, or whatever, and I said I can't relate to getting beat on or none of that, but I can relate to being in foster, we're all in foster care. That's what I said, you can relate to that."
2. 486	JAMES	"Yeah, OK, then he . . ."
2. 487	MITCHELL	"Yeah, that's the only thing I can relate to."
2. 488	JAMES	"OK, there we go then."
2. 489	JAMES	"And then he was gonna say somethin' next. I mean, I see what Mitchell's sayin' that he can't relate to it, but he relates to being in the foster care system."
2. 490	COUNSELOR	"Well, I'd like to take this conversation now and I'd like Rick to say what he was gonna say before." DIRECTING to challenge individual behavior in context
2. 491	JAMES	"Yeah, that's what I was trying to say, but I kept on trying to saying stuff."
2. 492	COUNSELOR	"Well, right now it's Rick's turn." DIRECTING to challenge group behavior
2. 493	RICK	"All right. I can sorta relate to you because my dad was a alcoholic, you know, and a drug user and everything, and I got beat when I was a kid and then that's why I came, so I can see how you're feeling right now."

2. 494	WALLACE	"Yeah, that's what I'm sayin'."
2. 495	THOMAS	"—— beat up —— your parents?"
2. 496	COUNSELOR	"Just a minute, Wallace." *Not a counseling response, although the counselor is "directing" Thomas*
2. 497	WALLACE	"Right, alcoholics, and stuff, and I used to learn on it. I got into fights when I was a little kid, like seven and eight years old."
2. 498	THOMAS	"Oh, yeah."
2. 499	WALLACE	"That's when I got tooken out of the situation. And I was goin' around slashin' tires when I was a little kid, runnin' around Seattle slashin' tires."
2. 500	COUNSELOR	"And, Rick, how is that for you to be interrupted?" QUESTIONING to explore individual experience
2. 501	RICK	"I'm in a different group besides this one and I'm used to being interrupted, but and then if I got mad enough I'd approach the person in mind saying, 'Now I'd really like it if you don't interrupt next time,' and I would really like to see you try and ask me before he could go ahead and say it."
2. 502	COUNSELOR	"But you didn't feel that before when you were trying to talk?" QUESTIONING to challenge individual feeling
2. 503	RICK	"Uh-huh."
2. 504	WALLACE	"Nope. I'm kinda used to it. you know, try to get like a point out. Your parents like cut you off, because they're afraid that you're gonna go off and like break something or hurt somebody."
2. 505	COUNSELOR	"So, you feel that way in this group . . ." *Response interrupted; continued at 2.507*
2. 506	WALLACE	"Yeah."
2. 507	COUNSELOR	". . . sometimes, people are cutting you off just like them?" EMPATHIZING to acknowledge individual feeling
2. 508	WALLACE	"You know it's like driving a car, idiot cuts in front and you slam on your breaks almost hit the damn idiot."
2. 509	THOMAS	"I think that a when you get, people get used to being cut off, if I think. For somebody normal just getting cut off, it can make 'em feel bad sometimes, when you make 'em feel like . . . For somebody normal just getting cut off, it can make 'em feel bad sometimes, when you make 'em feel like . . ."
2. 510	COUNSELOR	"How do you feel about being cut off?" QUESTIONING to challenge individual feeling

2. 511	THOMAS	"It depends on what I'm saying. If I'm saying something that's really important to me, right? Like a somethin' like a my basketball game, or I got somethin' that's really important to me, and I'm tryin' to say somethin, and then your parent just turns around and walks away, or somethin', that makes me, that makes you feel sort of bad because their 'spose to be the ones that are there for you, you know?"
2. 512	COUNSELOR	"But, Thomas, how do you feel about being cut off in this group?" QUESTIONING to challenge individual feeling in context
2. 513	THOMAS	"Well, I haven't been cut off here."
2. 514	WALLACE	"Yeah, exactly our point."
2. 515 ⬆	COUNSELOR	"So, you two are getting cut off, so it's the group . . . so Thomas is cutting people off." PARAPHRASE to acknowledge subgroup behavior
2. 516	THOMAS	"Oh, these guys cut more off than . . ."
2. 517	JAMES	"I saw him tryin' to say some stuff, so it's like this guy's goin' next because . . ."
2. 518	ERIC	"Let's not argue about that, OK?"
2. 519	WALLACE	"You know, I'm used to getting cut off. I'm used to having people not listen to me. That's what I've been like the whole time, I'm not, this is like, first foster home I lived with, people are actually listening to me, sit down and talk to me, ask me what's wrong. Did you know, I used to be like, I go home, nobody to talk to, right? So I just keep it in, and I keep it in and I get like suspended or something, 'cause someone just like pissed me off, and I like take out my anger on them."
2. 520	THOMAS	"I used to do the same thing."
2. 521	COUNSELOR	"So, are you feeling angry in group at times, holding it in? People cutting you off?" QUESTIONING to challenge individual feeling in context
2. 522	Wallace	"Well, sometimes, I mean, yeah, sometimes it just makes me want to take this damn chair I'm sittin' in and throw it at 'em, people all cut me off."
2. 523	COUNSELOR	"Yeah. Do you feel that way right now?" QUESTIONING to challenge individual feeling with immediacy
2. 524	WALLACE	"No." (laughs)
2. 525	COUNSELOR	"No. What's it like to now be able to talk in group?" QUESTIONING to challenge individual experience in context

2. 526	WALLACE	"I dunno, it feels good. You get to get out what you wanna say."
2. 527	COUNSELOR	"So, it feels good to you to be able to talk to everybody?" EMPATHIZING to acknowledge individual feeling in context *In question form* *The assumption of the in context focus is that "everyone" is the same as "group."*
2. 528	WALLACE	"Yeah."
2. 529	ERIC	"Sometimes it does, I think, feel good to get stuff off your chest, you know."
2. 530	WALLACE	"I know, especially when you have something important to say, you know, like get the first two words out and then someone cuts you off, it's just like . . ."
2. 531	ERIC	"That really, that frustrates me . . ."
2. 532	WALLACE	"Yeah."
2. 533	COUNSELOR	"I'm curious if Rick, how about you, 'cause you were saying you were having the same problem in group?" QUESTIONING to explore individual feeling in context
2. 534	RICK	"Being interrupted?"
2. 535	COUNSELOR	"Uh-huh." *Not a counseling response*
2. 536	RICK	"Well, it's sorta hard to discuss it because . . ."
2. 537	COUNSELOR	"How does it feel to have the floor now?" QUESTIONING to challenge individual feeling with immediacy
2. 538	RICK	"Oh, good, 'cause I get a lot attention, lot of positive attention."
2. 539	WALLACE	"Please."
2. 540	COUNSELOR	"Uh-huh. So like having the positive attention in group?" EMPATHIZING to acknowledge individual feeling in contents *In question form*
2. 541	RICK	"'Cause I'm an attention seeker, so I usually do bad things to seek negative attention. But when I get positive attention like this, makes me feel very good."
2. 542	WALLACE	"You just don't know what to do 'cause you get so used to getting negative attention, you know, 'cause, when like a bad person, when he like gets in trouble, right, and when he goes home and like people like tell him that he did something right, its just kinda like makes him feel good. Sometime it just makes him say like whatever."

2. 543a 2. 543b	COUNSELOR	"Thomas, I noticed after we were talking about interrupting that you stopped participating in group so much. I was wondering what's going on?" GIVING FEEDBACK to acknowledge individual behavior in context QUESTIONING to challenge individual experience
2. 544	THOMAS	"Yeah, 'cause these guys wanna talk. The way they put out what they had to say makes you feel like you're really being rude, you know? Like do you treat people the way you wanna be treated, you know? So if they don't feel good that I'm interrupin' them, you know, it's not that hard for me to shut up for a couple minutes, you know?"
2. 545	COUNSELOR	"So you were giving them the respect that you want from the group?" QUESTIONING to acknowledge individual behavior in context
2. 546	THOMAS	"Yeah, 'cause a people tell me what comes around goes around so you know . . . If I treat this guy like a jerk, over here, the next time I see him, say he's having a party or somethin' and he gives pops to everybody, he might not give one to me because, you know, he's treating me like this punk, you know, being crappy."
2. 547	ERIC	"I wouldn't let you in my party . . ."
2. 548	THOMAS	"See what I mean, he wouldn't even let me in the party, you know."
2. 549	ERIC	"You treat somebody the way they treat you, pretty much."
2. 550	COUNSELOR	"So, it was really important for the two of them to be able to speak so that you could a . . ." PARAPHRASING to acknowledge individual experience
2. 551	THOMAS	"A yeah, sorta like I gotta, sorta like I got a habit, you know,"
2. 552	COUNSELOR	"A habit you have?" CLARIFYING to explore individual behavior
2. 553	THOMAS	"Yeah."
2. 554a 2. 554b	COUNSELOR	"Well, I'd like to change the focus of group for a second and . . . ■ ______________ ● ______________ ▼ ______________ I was wondering if we could talk about what it was like to be here today?" ■ ______________ ● ______________ ▼ ______________
2. 555	JAMES	"I felt another thing was kinda him too, is like a, you know, I was going on about, you know, trying to prove myself to other people, is like since I didn't have, you know, parents or somethin' to say, you know, you did a good job, so I really related to him with that."

2. 556	MITCHELL	"I learned from James like at the house sometimes like he like sometimes he'll like be real active, you know, he'll like real quiet sometimes. I like understand like why you do the things you do, like why you're so into football because you wanna get out there and prove somethin'. Before I thought, you know, he just wanted to show off. But now I understand that you have a goal in life and your goal's to succeed, you know, and let everybody see your talent. And before, you know, I didn't understand it as much, and now I do, and that, like, that helps me out a lot."
2. 557	THOMAS	"I think when a these two were saying that I interrupted them, you know? It's not just the part of being aware of interruptin' again. It's sorta helpful, you know. It's sorta good that they told me what they were feeling 'cause say they didn't say what they felt like, I would continue to interrupt them and then they could end up getting really, really mad."
2. 558	RICK	"Can I pass?"
2. 559	COUNSELOR	"Well, I guess it's up to the group." DIRECTING to challenge group behavior *This more than a statement of fact, it is the counselor challenging the group to make a decision. The "guess" makes it sound like a hunch, but it is more DIRECTING, that is, the counselor is telling the group to decide.*
2. 560	THOMAS	"You didn't learn nothin'?"
2. 561	WALLACE	"You didn't learn anything about anybody in this group?"
2. 562	RICK	"OK, never mind now."
2. 563	WALLACE	"Oh, come on now, I learned stuff about you . . ."
2. 564	RICK	"Never mind. Never mind." *Note this change in his behavior and how he expressed his anger toward Wallace.*
2. 565	THOMAS	"Ohhhhhh. Attitude."
2. 566	THOMAS	"Getting to the end."
2. 567	ERIC	"Say somethin'."
2. 568	WALLACE	"Come on, fight, fight."
2. 569	COUNSELOR	"How do you feel right now, Rick?" QUESTIONING to challenge individual feeling with immediacy
2. 570	ERIC	"Can we just be quiet and let him say somethin', you know?"
2. 571	WALLACE	"I am 'cause . . ."
2. 572	COUNSELOR	"Rick, do you feel you have something to say? OK." QUESTIONING to challenge individual feeling

2. 573	ERIC	"Spit it out, brother."
2. 574	RICK	"Wallace, I just really appreciate next time if you would let me think before and I'd like to see you do that next time."
2. 575	WALLACE	"Uh-huh."
2. 576	ERIC	"All right, there you go."
2. 577	RICK	"OK. . . . I learned that well, what I said before, like about I can relate to some people, in that we all can relate to each other."
2. 578	COUNSELOR	"OK." *Not a counseling response*
2. 579	ERIC	"Well, like I said before, also, it feels good to like get stuff off of your chest and know that there's other, like a lot of time people just think about themselves and they're not thinking about other people, and like this makes you stop and think about well, I got all these problems but their problems are worse, or they got problems too, you know? Makes you stop and think about other people, not think about yourself so much."
2. 580	COUNSELOR	"And that helped you?" QUESTIONING to explore individual feeling
2. 581	ERIC	"Yeah."
2. 582	ERIC	"Everybody said something so the group's pretty much 'sposed to be closed."
2. 583	COUNSELOR	"Right, I think we're closing group now. OK, group's over." CLOSING to acknowledge group experience

Suggested Identifications for Selected Counselor Responses

Videocassette Exercise 2: Group 2/Boys

NUMBER	RESPONSE, INTENT, FOCUS
2. 8	EMPATHIZING to acknowledge group feeling
2. 30	PARAPHRASING to acknowledge subgroup experience
2. 40	QUESTIONING to challenge group experience with immediacy in context
2. 75	QUESTIONING to challenge group experience in context
2. 169	QUESTIONING to challenge group behavior in context with immediacy
2. 223	NOTING A THEME to challenge group feeling in context
2. 298	QUESTIONING to challenge individual feeling in context
2. 334	QUESTIONING to challenge individual feeling in context
2. 344	QUESTIONING to challenge group feeling *With 2.334, the one-two punch*
2. 445	GIVING FEEDBACK to acknowledge individual experience in context
2. 554a	DIRECTING to challenge group experience
2. 554b	QUESTIONING to challenge group experience *Multiple responses*

Advanced Exercises

Advanced Exercises 1–5 are designed to be done with an actual group in which the student demonstrates counseling responses in the group. The exercises are developmental, each exercise building on the previous one. As in all counselor training situations, professional supervision is suggested because these exercises require student-to-client interaction. The purpose of these exercises is to become familiar with what a group counselor might say, although students may initially feel awkward and artificially demonstrate counseling responses. It is expected that with time and further training, students will not only feel more comfortable and confident but will use responses that are therapeutically appropriate.

Set up a group, whether it be an actual group or simulated group. The group should have at least six members. Try to arrange a consistent group that can meet at least five times. A minimum of 60 minutes per session is suggested.

Advanced Exercise 1

Demonstrate

Videotape a group session. Discuss confidentiality. Practice using the *essential* responses of OPENING OR CLOSING and ATTENDING, plus other appropriate counseling responses.

Observe

View the video.

Identify

Use the Counselor Response Identification Form (CRIF) in Appendix A to identify as many counseling RESPONSES and respective intents and focuses as possible.

Reflect

1. Describe the experience of viewing yourself as a group counselor in the videotaped session.
2. Describe what was seen on the video that was not observed during the session.

Advanced Exercise 2

Demonstrate

Videotape a group session. Demonstrate as many of the following *passive* responses as possible: EMPATHIZING, PARAPHRASING, and GIVING FEEDBACK.

Observe

View the video.

Identify

Use the CRIF in Appendix A to identify as many counseling RESPONSES and respective intents and focuses as possible.

Reflect

1. Discuss age, gender, ethnic, and other relevant client and counselor variables and how they may influence the group dynamics.
2. Describe the stage development of the group at this point.

Advanced Exercise 3

Demonstrate

Videotape a group session. Demonstrate any of the *active* responses of CLARIFYING, DIRECTING, and QUESTIONING; plus the *discretionary* responses of ALLOWING SILENCE and SELF-DISCLOSING. Use other responses as appropriate.

Observe

View the video.

Identify

Use the CRIF in Appendix A to identify as many counseling RESPONSES and respective intents and focuses as possible.

Reflect

1. Describe the stage development of the group at this point.
2. Define any challenges or issues that, as a group counselor, you are experiencing at this time.

Advanced Exercise 4

Demonstrate

Videotape a group session. Use appropriate counseling responses, keeping the focus on the GROUP as much as possible. Try to use immediacy. Include, if possible, at least one of the *interpretive* responses: PLAYING A HUNCH, NOTING A THEME, NOTING A DISCREPANCY, NOTING A CONNECTION, and REFRAMING.

Observe

View the video.

Identify

Use the CRIF in Appendix A to identify as many counseling RESPONSES and respective intents and focuses as possible.

Reflect

1. Describe the stage development of the group at this point.
2. What might be expected to happen in the next group session, and what plans might you have to respond to this?

Advanced Exercise 5

Demonstrate

Videotape a group session. Before the group starts, identify specific RESPONSES with associated intents and focuses that can be used in the group. Pay special attention to this being the last session of the group.

Observe

View the video.

Identify

Use the CRIF in Appendix A to identify as many counseling RESPONSES and respective intents and focuses as possible.

Reflect

1. What responses were used in this group to give time for processing termination?
2. Name any ethical and diversity issues that arose during this or other group sessions. Discuss your response to these issues.
3. Name specific counseling responses, intents, and focuses that seem to work best for you as a group counselor.
4. What have you learned about being a group counselor from these advanced exercises?

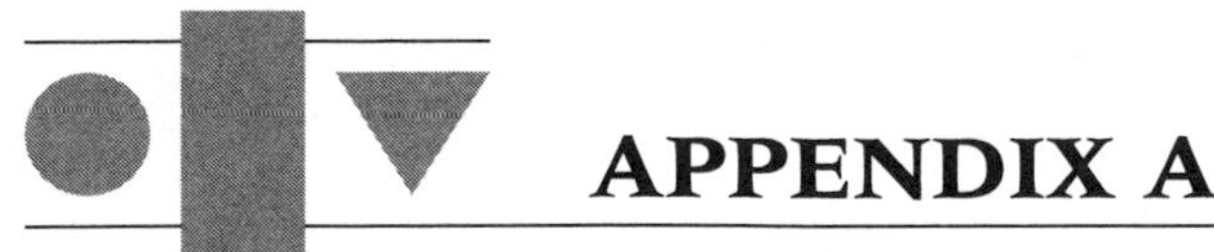

APPENDIX A

Counseling Response Identification Format (CRIF) for Videocassette Exercises 1 and 2
Counseling Response Identification Format (CRIF) for Advanced Exercises 1–5
Examples of Individual Goals
Confidentiality Transcript: Group 5/Adults
Diagrams of Groups
Charts 1–5: Frequency of "I," "You," "We" Usage
Chart 6: Use of Counseling Responses by Clients
Transcript of Group 3/Graduates
Transcript of Group 4/Students
Transcript of Group 5/Adults
Follow-up of Group Clients
Table 1: Comparing *Basic Counseling Reponses in Groups* to Responses/Skills of Other Models
Figures 1, 2, and 3: Response, Intent, and Focus

Basic Counseling Responses in Groups

Counseling Response Indentification Format (CRIF)
for
Videocassette Exercises 1 and 2

Student ______________________________ Counselor response ____________
____

■ Response	● Intent	▼ Focus
☐ Opening or closing ☐ Attending ☐ Empathizing ☐ Paraphrasing ☐ Giving feedback ☐ Questioning ☐ Clarifying ☐ Directing ☐ Playing a hunch ☐ Noting a theme ☐ Noting a discrepancy ☐ Noting a connection ☐ Reframing ☐ Allowing silence ☐ Self-disclosing	☐ Acknowledge ☐ Explore ☐ Challenge ⇦ Check a response; For multiple or combination responses, number each response. ⇨ There can be multiple "whats." ⇨ One or both additives are in addition to a "who" or "what."	*Who* ☐ Group ☐ Subgroup ☐ Individual *What* ☐ Experience ☐ Thought ☐ Feeling ☐ Behavior Additives (optional) *Where* ☐ Context *When* ☐ Immediacy

Basic Counseling Responses in Groups

Counseling Response Indentification Format (CRIF)
for
Advanced Exercises 1–5

Student ______________________ Group __________ Session __________

Verbatim interaction between clients(s) and counselor

Client (name) ____

Counselor ____

Client (name) ____

■ Response

- ☐ Opening or closing
- ☐ Attending
- ☐ Empathizing
- ☐ Paraphrasing
- ☐ Giving feedback
- ☐ Questioning
- ☐ Clarifying
- ☐ Directing
- ☐ Playing a hunch
- ☐ Noting a theme
- ☐ Noting a discrepancy
- ☐ Noting a connection
- ☐ Reframing
- ☐ Allowing silence
- ☐ Self-disclosing

● Intent

- ☐ Acknowledge
- ☐ Explore
- ☐ Challenge

⇦ Check a response; For multiple or combination responses, number each response.

⇨ There can be multiple "whats."

⇨ One or both additives are in addition to a "who" or "what."

▼ Focus

Who

- ☐ Group
- ☐ Subgroup
- ☐ Individual

What

- ☐ Experience
- ☐ Thought
- ☐ Feeling
- ☐ Behavior

Additives

Where

- ☐ Context

When

- ☐ Immediacy

Examples of Individual Goals

Clients who volunteered for groups 1, 3, and 5 were asked to submit written goals of what they wanted from the group counseling experience. The following are examples of those submissions:

- To learn better ways to handle the stress of being in school, working, and having a social life. To gain more insight into how the stress of my responsibilities affects my interpersonal relationships.
- Work to positively engage with others who are part of the graduate student experience and decrease my sense of isolation. I also want to work to examine my own thoughts and feelings and behaviors when engaged with others to gain some insight about myself in relation to particular kinds of people. Be honest and open.
- I'd like to work on being more able to take risks, being more able to speak my mind, and being more relaxed when speaking or presenting in front of strangers.
- To increase the extent to which I share my inner thoughts and feelings. My second goal is to improve my attentiveness to others.
- My goals for a group of women discussing life issues are parenting adult children and transitioning to middle age.
- I want to discuss with other women thoughts about aging and changing familiar roles, and the feelings that occur in the process. I want support from others to know that I can make this transition, see the humor in it, and get ideas on how to care for myself.
- To work on developing a relationship with my brother based on what is possible, not on what should or ought to be . . . working towards acceptance of our individual situations, letting go of guilt that is not useful. To come to understand and feel that I am not entirely responsible for his condition.
- I would love to work on body image, self-esteem, and quitting smoking.
- I'd like to use the group to explore why I have pulled back from any kind of community involvement and to look at what is keeping me from investing in other activities.
- I would like to discuss my experience of being a new father and the developmental issues around this. I could also talk about the stresses on my relationship with my spouse during this new life phase.
- Have an opportunity to talk about life after graduation. Where will we work? Job opportunities? Interview tips? Tips for coping with the stress of graduate school. What are some ways people manage their time? How do they balance school and life outside of it?
- Explore why it's hard to make friends in the counseling program. It's hard to get to know people outside of class. Why is this?
- I would like to learn coping skills, not survival techniques. Other issues include feelings of stress and isolation relative to the demands of school.
- I would like to gain a better understanding of how I react to different individuals in a group setting. I would like to communicate what is on my mind rather than sit there and let my thoughts go unheard and unexpressed. I would like to take more initiative and be more expressive rather than letting people assume that they can read what is going on inside of my head.
- I would like to use this group encounter to experiment with a support group of other graduate students. I would like to explore my own experience as a graduate student against the background of others' experiences. I would hope to gain energy and self-understanding from participating in this group.

- I would like to gain a better understanding of my values and beliefs and how they will play a role in becoming a secondary school counselor.
- To gain some insight/knowledge about my relationships. I would like to explore why I have such difficulties beginning and sustaining relationships with men and why I have had such a difficult time in starting new relationships since I have moved to Seattle in the last few years.
- To continue to learn more about myself as I relate both to myself and to others around me. One way in which I'd like to learn more about myself is in relation to how I handle stress.
- To develop personal competency in problem management through peer interaction. To identify common life issues with my peers and participate in group analysis related to these issues. To develop greater insight regarding areas for personal development.
- I plan to be open to the experience and to give honest feedback to the other members.
- My goal for the group would be to try to figure out what I can do and/or what prevents me from making time for myself.
- I feel that my emotional state is relatively flat. I would like to enjoy my emotional highs more than I currently do. I want to explore this aspect of myself in a group setting.

Confidentiality Transcript: Group 5/Adults

The following transcript is of a discussion on confidentiality by Group 5/adults. This discussion is not on the videocassette or the CD-ROM.

COUNSELOR A: Confidentiality is something we usually talk about at the beginning of a group. Meaning that what we say here stays here or it won't go outside this group. Often that's something that makes people feel more comfortable. It makes me feel more comfortable to know if I say something to you about myself I am only saying it to you and it's not going to be passed on to other people I might know somewhere else. And that is a norm that we establish in our groups; that is, what we say here will stay here.

CAROL: Thank you for saying that because I was really concerned about that because although I don't see this as being necessarily really, you know, provocative in terms of the things that we talk about but, but I think that it makes it a little bit easier to be honest about what's on my mind.

MATT: What I'm doing also is . . . reminding myself that we are all here for similar areas . . . if not the same reason. You know we're all here to get something out of this experience. That kinda helps me with being willing to be open with the group and, and, and share about myself, because we all are here to . . . get something out it, out of the experience, so.

COUNSELOR A: You aren't the only one who wants to reveal something . . .

MATT: Right, yeah.

KEVIN: I can say a little bit more about that, to the confidentiality . . . it is a really big value for me . . . in my own personal life with my friends and family. It is important to me to be able to have my family's confidence and my friends'. . . . I like to know that I can trust a person when I'm talking about something that is meaningful to me. So, in this group, you know, I would like to feel that whatever I say is being held confidence and that the people I am talking to will respect what I'm saying and what I'm feeling.

COUNSELOR A: So, trust to you means . . .?

KEVIN: Trust, and I guess I put them side by side, trust and confidence.

COUNSELOR A: OK.

KEVIN: . . . It's important to me to be able to have a person's confidence, but at the same time, or at the same time, I like to be able to trust a person, or know that I can trust a person to keep my confidence. So, I guess they go together.

COUNSELOR A: Um-hmm.

SHELLEY: I would agree with that. I have . . . It's really important for me to know that other people feel that they can trust me with information or just with whatever they would want to share and . . . That is something that I value and so . . . and I know that that doesn't just come. You can't just tell someone that you can trust them with anything. But . . . but, I'd like to . . . I don't know. I guess that is hard to do in a, in a . . . when you first meet people, how that develops, but . . . but just to feel like . . . that I can be trusted with information and then to as well be able to share things and know that its not going to go anywhere inappropriate. I guess. Well, I think that I worry less about other people talking about my stuff than I do about just making sure that I'm being trustworthy.

COUNSELOR A: Two sides to it.

SHELLEY: Yeah, yeah there are.

COUNSELOR B: So, I just want to make sure . . . So, for you it's important that other people know that they can trust what they say with you.

SHELLEY: Yeah. Yeah.

COUNSELOR B: OK. It is not so much that you worry about you. Keeping it . . . as you want to make sure that other people know and you want to communicate the fact that, yeah, you can trust me and it will go no farther than this. It's not going to go into the next town and it stops here.

SHELLEY: Right. Right.

COUNSELOR A: So, I notice we are finding common agreement that we want to trust, and we're all agreeing that trust is important and that . . . it would be hard to take a risk that if we don't trust . . . and aren't we trustworthy.

COUNSELOR B: And one of the things that may engender that trust is that everybody insist, discloses kinda, where they are at the present time. That's kinda what I heard Carol saying. It made you a little more relaxed to hear that other people were also anxious and . . . kinda sharing where they are and not kinda holding back.

CAROL: Uh-huh. Definitely.

Diagrams of Groups

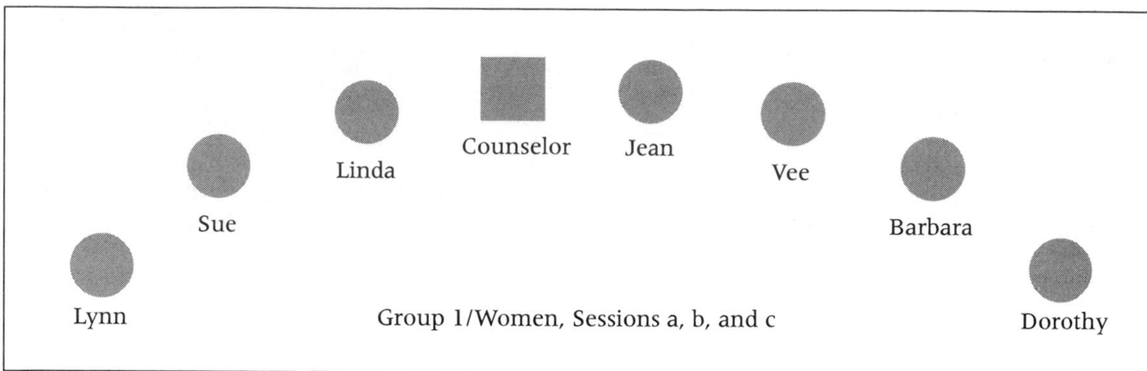

Group 1/Women, Sessions a, b, and c

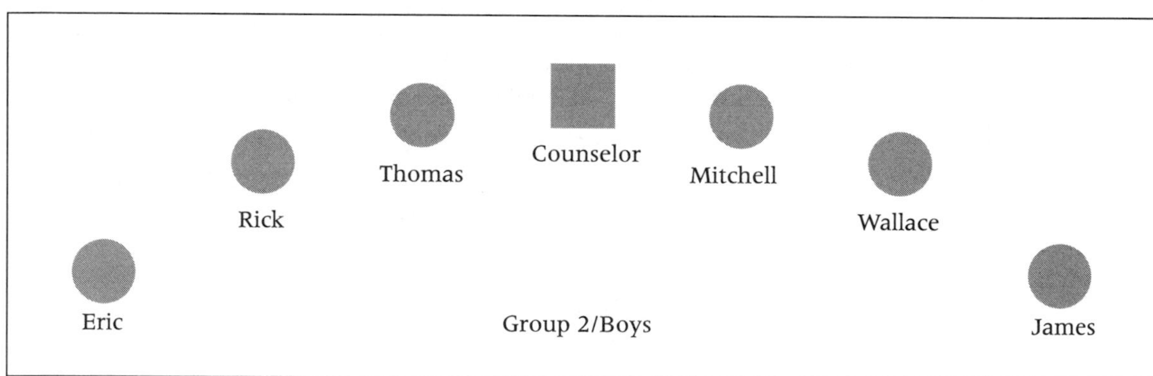

Group 2/Boys

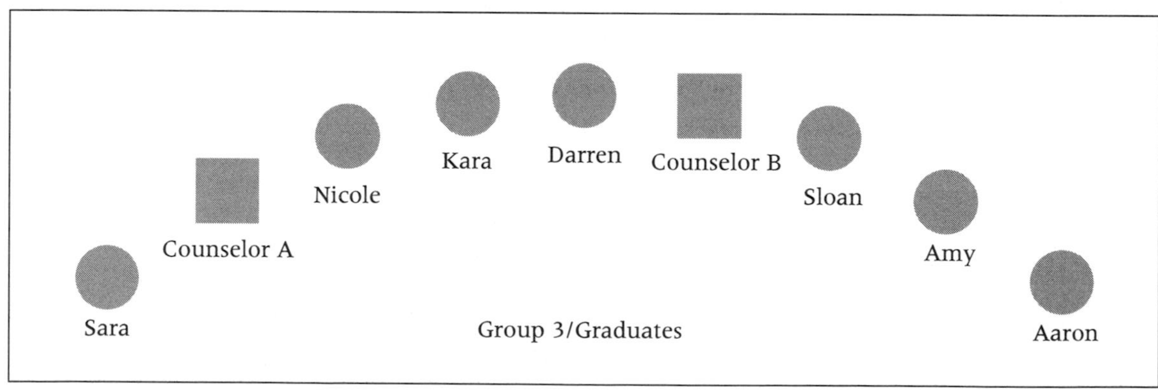

Group 3/Graduates

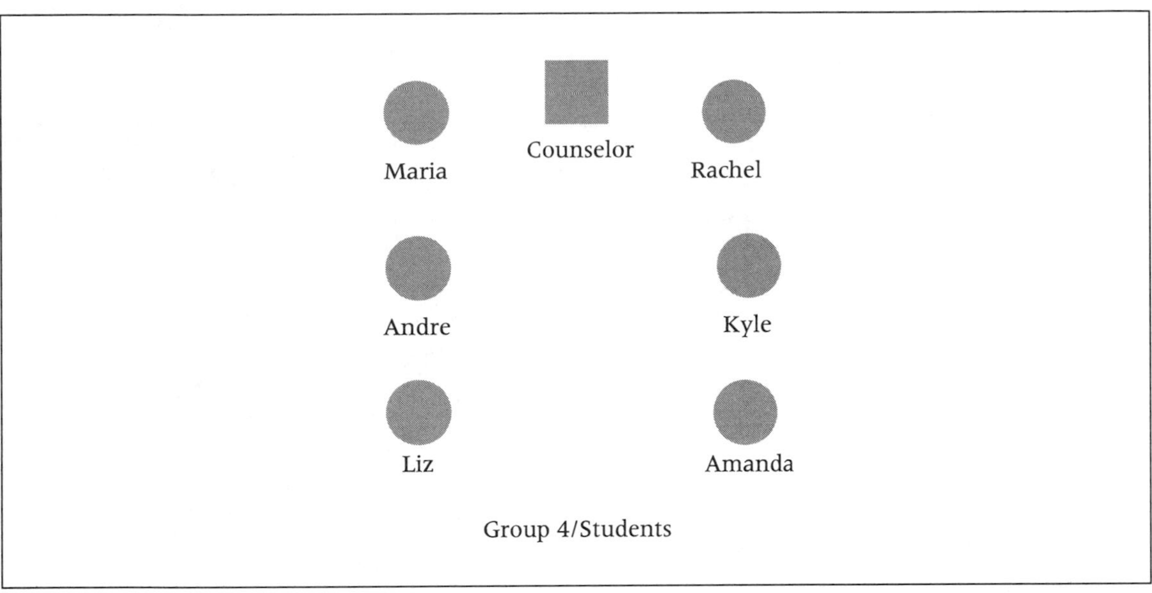

Group 4/Students

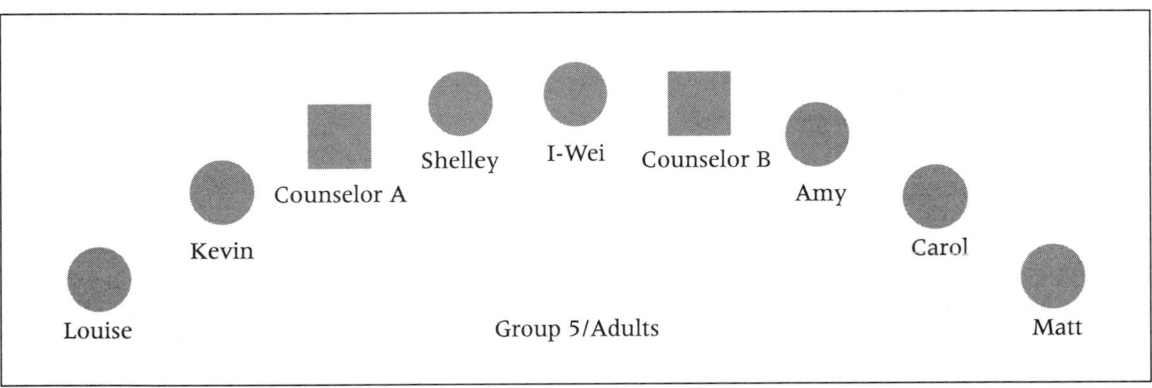

Group 5/Adults

CHART 1 Group 1/Women: Frequency of "I," "You," "We" Usage

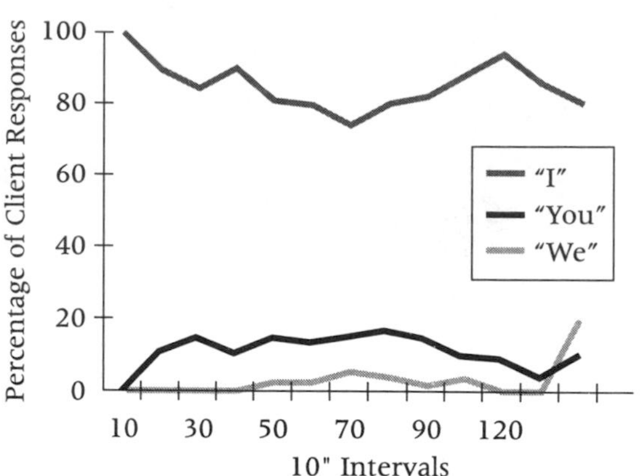

CHART 2 Group 2/Boys: Frequency of "I," "You," "We" Usage

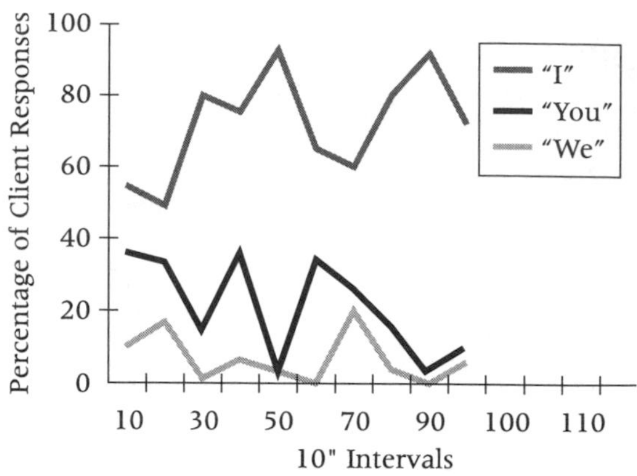

CHART 3 Group 3/Graduates: Frequency of "I," "You," "We" Usage

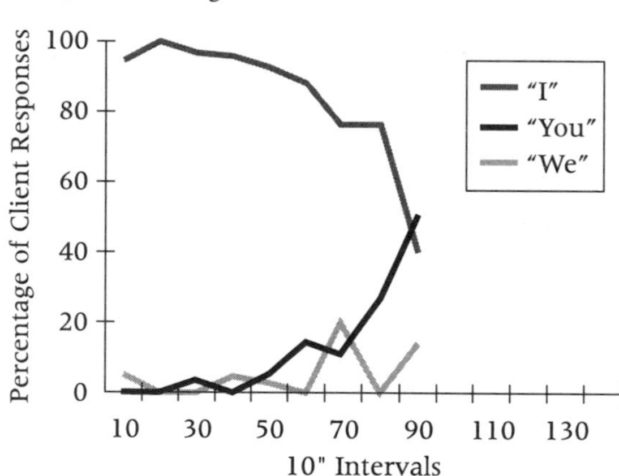

CHART 4 Group 4/Students: Frequency of "I," "You," "We" Usage

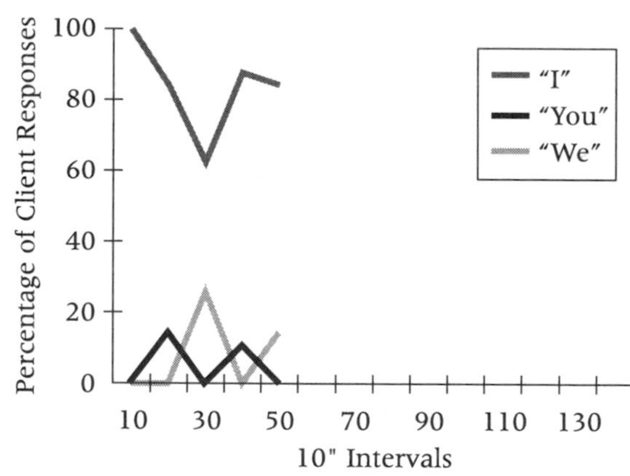

CHART 5 Group 5/Adults: Frequency of "I," "You," "We" Usage

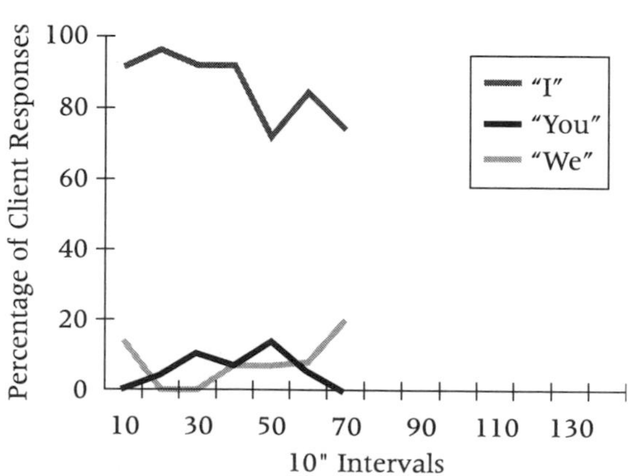

CHART 6 Use of Counseling Responses by Clients

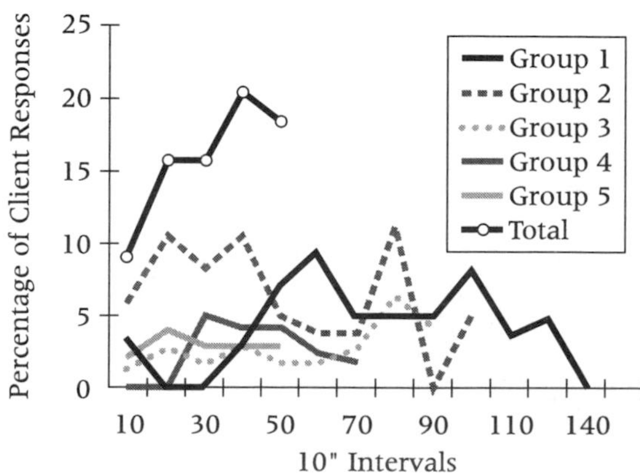

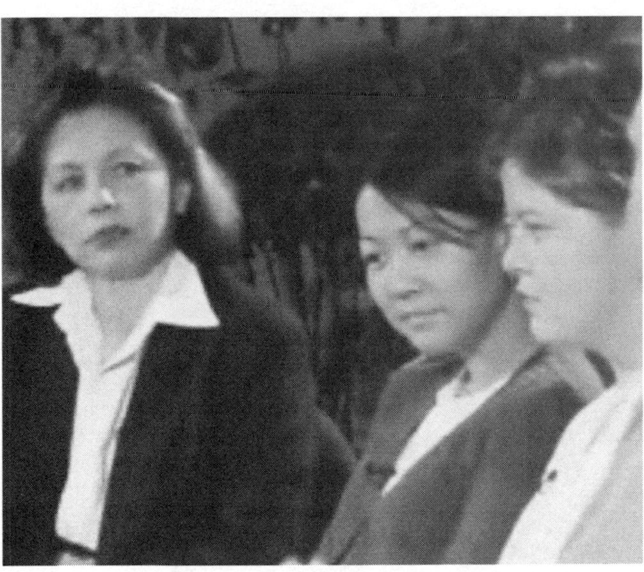

Transcript of Group 3/Graduates

3. 1	COUNSELOR B	"How would the group like to start?" OPENING to acknowledge group experience
3. 2	DARREN	"Well, I was thinking that one thing that I, kind of self-analyzing, um, because as I say, probably about the last three or four months I've been experiencing this kind of flatness of emotion. Not that I don't have happy times and sad times, but it just doesn't last that long. And pretty soon I'm back to this 'I'm going through this internship, I'm going through graduate school, when will it be over?' type of thing and that's been bothering me. But, I, you know, its been a period throughout the winter. I don't know, it may be just the weather has been so bad that that's been why. That's what's been going through my head. Maybe it's just the weather, maybe that's why I'm just kind of in this blasé mood."
3. 3	AARON	"I mean, I felt that way last quarter and the first quarter of my internship a lot and I think now that I'm in my third quarter and that's really getting near the end I feel that that blasé mood has gone up a lot. I know like last quarter I was just completely down in the dumps and hated everything and was convinced that I was the worst counselor ever and that I should just get out of this field immediately and so forth. But I think now that it's just, that I have a month left, almost 5 weeks, the mood just kind of naturally picks up."

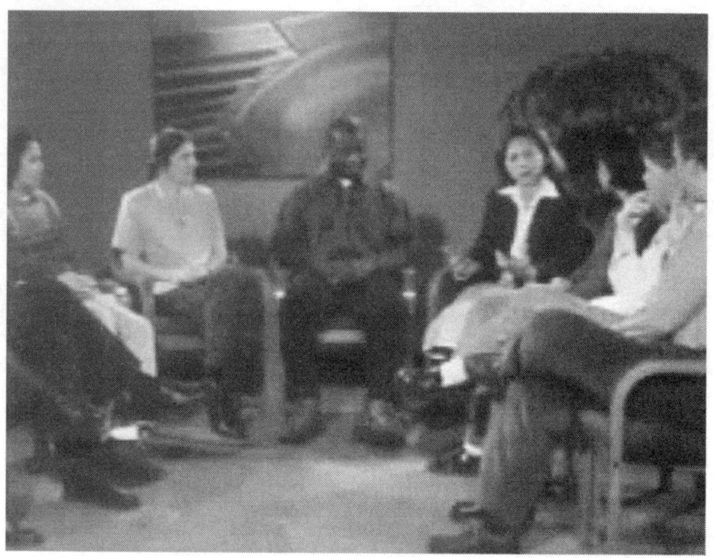

3. 4	COUNSELOR B	"I also heard a theme of maybe disenchantment or kind of now we're here, we've gone through this and you know, what if I don't really like what I'm doing. That's kind of something that I heard." NOTING A THEME to challenge group experience
3. 5	AMY	"That's a huge, huge fear of mine. Huge. Um, I could go on for hours. Yeah, because you start out and you're learning new things and it's exciting. And it is like I, this is going to sound silly, it's like you're going to run a road race and you start out at the beginning, the start of the first quarter, it is an excited kind of energy. Then in the middle, it's like I wondered why I ever even started this. And now I'm at the end and I'm thinking I'm just gonna do what I gotta do to get to the end. And now I'm working hard to get to the end and now I'm not so sure that I like what I can see past the old, 'You're finished' sign. Yeah, so that's bothersome to not know . . . You know, I mean, we've been working hard and to not know if that's all been worth it, and plus I'm just tired and so I think that that lends to being disenchanted and dissatisfied and whatever else, so."
3. 6	NICOLE	"I can agree with that. It seems to me like I am always trying to start new things and try to get some change brought about. We're moving into a new school next year, and you know it seems to me like we don't want to bring the same problems up there. I want to start new things, but yet everybody else is just kind of at this stuck point, and we just can't seem to get anywhere, and, then, it's frustrating because you, you know, you're trying to bring in all this energy and you just can't seem to get anywhere."

3. 7	AMY	"And maybe that's my problem is that it's getting a little frustrating talking about taking all these things from here and then applying it to the real world. It doesn't always work as nicely as one would hope."
3. 8a 3. 8b	COUNSELOR A	"I've noticed several members talking about feeling frustrated with what's going on as part of their education or personal lives." PARAPHRASING to acknowledge subgroup feeling "I am wondering if other people are feeling frustrated about what's happening here, right now?" QUESTIONING to challenge subgroup experience with immediacy in context
3. 9	NICOLE	"Sometimes it's kind of nice to hear that other people may have frustrations, not necessarily here but outside, that you're not the only one because sometimes you're just going, 'Am I the only one that is feeling, you know, overwhelmed or frustrated?' So it's nice to know other people are having some of those thoughts as well."
3. 10	KARA	"Yeah, I definitely agree. I think that often times we get caught up in, or at least I get caught up in school, and work, and then it's easy to think, 'Gosh, I'm alone. Am I alone in this? Is anyone else experiencing this kind of frustration?' Or just wanting to, you know, just leave for an hour, just, you know, kind of take a step out of it."
3. 11a 3. 11b	COUNSELOR B	"I kinda wanted to circle back to how this experience is for you right now . . . DIRECTING to challenge group experience . . . I heard the word *frustration.*" GIVING FEEDBACK to acknowledge group behavior
3. 12	AMY	"My thing is that we are sitting here talking about all of the challenges in our life, and my intent was not to come here and be challenged. Does that make sense? 'Cause I think I mean talking about the deeper stuff and whatever, whether it is sadness or disappointment or semantics, I don't know. But it feels challenging, and I didn't want to come here and be challenged. I wanted to come here and be whiny and supported. So I guess that explains my frustration."
3. 13	SLOAN	"It is like another demand being put on us. The members want to talk about something and then, you know, the counselors are saying . . . you know, pulling us in a different direction and then it's distracting and, you know, it may be taking away some of that energy that the members were going on."

3. 14	COUNSELOR B	"I was wondering if there is a connection between the feeling that the group has about the demands that Martin and I put on the group and also the frustration you are feeling with the demands of the outside upon you at this point." NOTING A CONNECTION to challenge group feeling
3. 15	AMY	"I think there's a connection. Um. I don't know how to explain this. I think, well, I'll speak for myself. I often have to be challenged to do something that I may not at the moment appreciate a whole lot in order to greatly appreciate when it is all over. Does that make sense? So, and as far as outside this group, um, I'm losing my train of thought. It's not fun right now, but I think that when it is all over I will very much appreciate the experience and I will be glad when it's done, and I will have more choices and it will be a good thing. And I think it's very similar to right now. Maybe I don't want to go your direction because it isn't very fun to go wherever it is we are trying to go, but it's maybe where we need to go. I don't know. Now I'm just going on and on, I'll stop now."
3. 16a 3. 16b	COUNSELOR A	"It seems like Lupe and I keep on trying to bring in discussions about what's happening on the outside of this room right now, in and it keeps going out . . . GIVING FEEDBACK to challenge group behavior . . . I'm wondering what that's about, what people's hunches are." QUESTIONING to challenge group thought
3. 17	AARON	"I almost feel like, it's uncomfortable for the counselors and that you're doing something that you feel uncomfortable with being in the group. And, it feels like, I am almost feeling more frustration from you two about us going our way and vice versa."
3. 18	COUNSELOR A	"Well, you know, when you say that I think to myself, I think, I do have a bias that I bring into here and that is, usually when I've done other groups like this is, what is important to people are their relationships and I kinda expected you to talk about maybe the impact your school was having on your relationships and not where you want to go. So maybe I am guilty of kinda leading you in that direction 'cause maybe that's where I want you to go." SELF-DISCLOSING to challenge group experience
3. 19	AARON	"I really appreciate you saying that, Martin."
3. 20	COUNSELOR B	"The frustration, just to address what Aaron said, that I'm feeling right now . . . I have a sense that . . . it seems to me we shifted again, and that's part of my frustration." SELF-DISCLOSING to acknowledge group experience with immediacy

3. 21	COUNSELOR A	"So, how was it for the group to hear that Lupe and I were frustrated also?" QUESTIONING to challenge group experience
3. 22	NICOLE	"Well, I think it's good, you know, that we hear sometimes how both of you are feeling because it makes things seem more real. That you are here, and you're listening to what, you know, we're saying."
3. 23	AARON	"I feel like in a way it is accomplishing what she wanted for us to accomplish and that's to talk about what we're feeling in the group."
3. 24	AMY	"I have to be honest and say that it's good for me to hear a different perspective, but although I have to admit, the fact that you guys are frustrated means less to me than if these guys were frustrated."

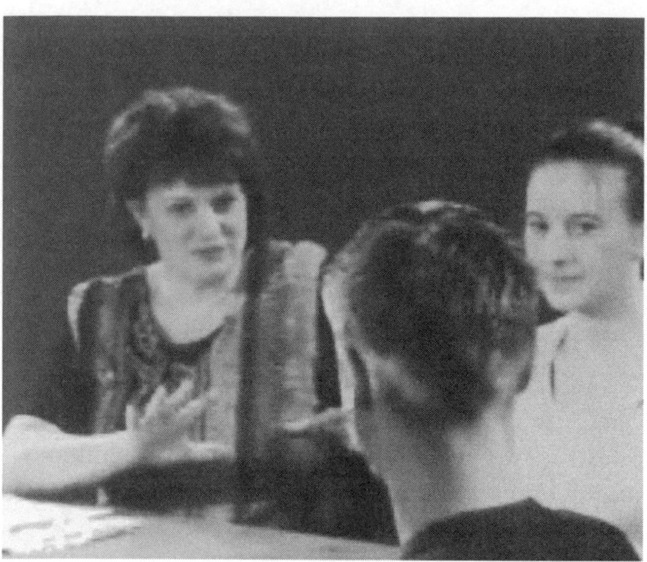

Transcript of Group 4/Students

4. 1a 4. 1b	COUNSELOR	"Last week we spent a little time getting to know each other and today what I would like to do is see the group start with a check in. And a check in is 'where are you?' Where are you? You know it is 3rd period today and it's Monday, but where are you at? So I would like if you could take just a minute to think about this and then you can check in as you feel you'd like to start. And basically check in was, would be, 'I'm feeling . . .' and then you can put in what feeling how you are doing today and the reason why, because. DIRECTING to challenge group experience So for example, I could say if I would be checking in and which I'd like to check in, I would say I'm feeling rushed today because this is the first day of the semester and I had a lot of schedule changes to make. So today I'm checking in and saying I'm feeling rushed today." SELF-DISCLOSING to acknowledge individual experience *Note that this was done to model checking in for the group clients.*
4. 2	KYLE	"All eyes are on me . . . I don't know. Today, I'm just cool, just laid back, 'cause I'm not doing nothing, so I'm all right."
4. 3	COUNSELOR	"OK, just laid back and relaxed." PARAPHRASING to acknowledge individual experience
4. 4	MARIA	"I'm feeling tired because it is Monday."

4. 5	ANDRE	"I'm also kinda tired because I stayed up late last night watching TV."
4. 6	MARIA	"What's on Sundays, I don't know."
4. 7	RACHEL	"I'm feeling really slowed down, because first period was kind of boring for me and I just started my day being really slow."
4. 8	MARIA	"I agree."
4. 9	LIZ	"I'm feeling kinda mad and sad because last night my mom and I got into a fight about something."
4. 10	COUNSELOR	"All right." ATTENDING to acknowledge individual experience *This is an example of a verbal ATTENDING response.*
4. 11	AMANDA	"Today has been good so far, but I'm just really tired because I stayed up late last night too."
4. 12a	COUNSELOR	"So I notice that two people are basically tired because they had stayed up late . . ." GIVING FEEDBACK to acknowledge subgroup feeling
4. 12b		". . . Before we move on to talking about what we said we were going to talking about some anger, can we stop here for just a minute? . . . DIRECTING to challenge group behavior
4. 12c		. . . and Kyle, you just shared something that when there was sort of a silence you were saying that people sort of turn to you." PARAPHRASING to acknowledge individual behavior
4. 12d		"Did you feel that when, that people look to you to start something or to be the leader?" QUESTIONING to challenge individual behavior
4. 13	KYLE	"Well, when it comes to a lot of things, sometimes. Yeah."
4. 14	COUNSELOR	"Can you explain a little bit more about that?" CLARIFYING to explore individual behavior
4. 15	KYLE	"Well, I don't know, 'cause, for instance, basketball. All of the coaches are looking at me because I'm telling people what to do. It just naturally . . . I know what to do without anybody having to tell me."
4. 16	COUNSELOR	"Does anyone here in this group notice that they look to Kyle to maybe start things out?" QUESTIONING to challenge group behavior
4. 17	RACHEL	"I don't usually, like, look to anyone. I kinda try to be independent and do stuff on my own. But, like, in 1st period if I'm in a

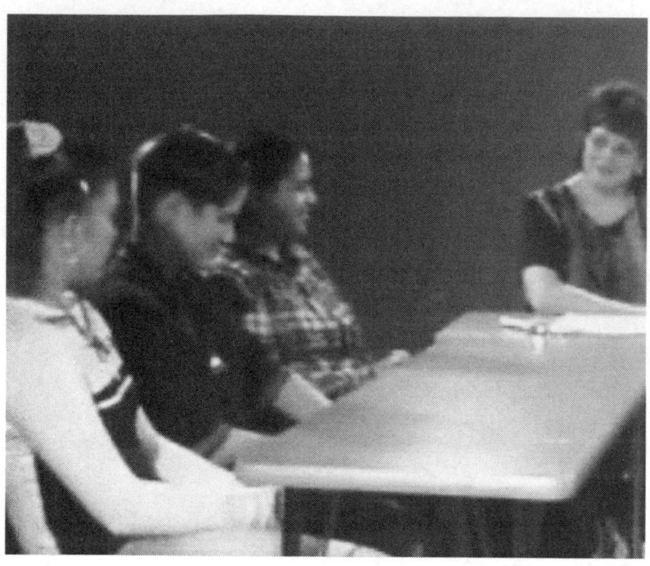

		group with Kyle he just usually, naturally, before I even have a chance to like do, like try to be the leader, or something, he just kinda takes charge and it works out."
4. 18a	MARIA	"But most of the time, sometimes, people don't agree with him and he can't accept it."
4. 19	KYLE	"I like to prove my point if I feel that I'm right, ain't that right?"
4. 20	COUNSELOR	"Kyle, you sort of got put on the spot by just your check in. What about if we just stand back for a second. How does it feel to get some feedback from Rachel about . . . ?" QUESTIONING to challenge individual feeling
4. 21	KYLE	"I get feedback from her all the time."
4. 22	COUNSELOR	"How did it feel to hear the feedback from Rachel that in 1st period you do stand out as a leader?" QUESTIONING to challenge individual behavior
4. 23	KYLE	"I don't know. It's just, yeah, it was nice to know."
4. 24	MARIA	"I think he feels put on the spot again."
4. 25	COUNSELOR	"Is that something you wanted to ask him, or is that just a hunch you have?" QUESTIONING to challenge individual behavior
4. 26	MARIA	"I don't know. It just felt like it."

4. 27	RACHEL	"Sometimes people just agree with him because they are afraid to have their own opinions. 'Cause I mean, sometimes Kyle can be kinda intimidating, and I mean, I don't mean that in a bad way, but sometimes he just proves his point and makes it sound like that's all that there can be so, um, sometimes they are just so intimidated they just agree with him even though they don't really believe what he is saying."
4. 28	KYLE	"Really? Wow! I had no idea!"
4. 29	COUNSELOR	"How does that sound to say that some people are agreeing because they're . . ." QUESTIONING to challenge individual experience
4. 30	KYLE	"I don't find myself very intimidating. I mean . . ."
4. 31	COUNSELOR	"So your perception, I'm sorry I interrupted . . ." *Not a complete response*
4. 32	KYLE	"People get afraid of me because they think I flunked like, four times. Oh, well, it's not my problem. It gives me an advantage."
4. 33	COUNSELOR	"So the intimidation can give you an advantage?" PARAPHRASING to acknowledge individual experience *In question form*
4. 34	KYLE	"Yeah, like, I walked into my first basketball game this season, and you hear like five people say, 'There's the guy from Nelson with a beard.' They get scared."
4. 35	MARIA	"I think your sideburns are the things that scare people. It's just unusual."
4. 36	COUNSELOR	"You changed what you said from scaring people to just unusual." GIVING FEEDBACK to acknowledge individual behavior
4. 37	MARIA	"It's just like, different, I don't know. He's the only person in the school with sideburns."
4. 38a 4. 38b	COUNSELOR	"We have been looking at Kyle quite a bit, and people are making some assumptions just looking at him." PARAPHRASING to acknowledge group behavior "Are any, is anyone else in this group . . . do people make assumptions about you because of how you look or how you speak up?" QUESTIONING to challenge group experience
4. 39	MARIA	"Well, once in a while, sometimes people think, I don't know, they just automatically think that I am like, black, or they just say that I'm Mexican or something and nobody ever asks me and it really

		just makes me mad. 'Cause they just always like . . . Like whenever like a subject comes up, like doing our hair or something, and they don't understand and they're just like, 'Well, you have black hair' or something and I don't."
4. 40	KYLE	"Well, one time I commented that you were Ethiopian and you hit me! You just slugged me."
4. 41	MARIA	"No, 'cause you didn't say 'Ethiopian' you said 'Ethe,' and that really made me angry."
4. 42	KYLE	"I didn't say 'Ethe.'"
4. 43	MARIA	"You don't want me to call you 'whitey'!"
4. 44	KYLE	"I don't care though."
4. 45	MARIA	"Well, I do care."
4. 46	KYLE	"OK."
4. 47	MARIA	"And the vice principal thought that I was Mexican. And she was like saying all this stuff to me about how about something about getting a job or something (laughs) . . . And me being Hispanic and how it's not going to get me anywhere in the world, and I was like, 'Well, actually I am mixed.' And she's like, 'No you're not.' My mom had to tell her and then she believed me, and it made me angry."
4. 48	COUNSELOR	"But what I'm hearing you say is that we don't need to guess, and that if we have a question we can ask." PARAPHRASING to acknowledge individual experience in context
4. 49	MARIA	"I wouldn't care if people ask me. They always just assume nobody ever asks me."
4. 50	COUNSELOR	"What are some of your reactions to what Maria just shared?" QUESTIONING to challenge group experience
4. 51	ANDRE	"I guess you shouldn't just assume stuff about people before you know them. You should, like, get to know them."
4. 52	COUNSELOR	"Can you restate that with 'I' with what message you got, Andre?" DIRECTING to challenge individual behavior
4. 53	ANDRE	"Like, if I don't know something about somebody, I shouldn't think that it is true. I shouldn't just assume that it's true without like positively knowing that it is true."
4. 54	KYLE	"Like if you're not going to know, you should just ask 'em."

4. 55a 4. 55b	COUNSELOR	"One other thing came up in check in, and Liz, you had said that today was a hard day for you, I can't remember what feeling you gave." PARAPHRASING to acknowledge individual experience "Do you remember the feeling you gave with check in?" QUESTIONING to explore individual feeling
4. 56	LIZ	"I was sad and mad and had mixed feelings. My mom and I got in a argument about me going over to my friend's house because there was going to be no adult there, and I think that she should have some trust in me, you know, and not assume that I'm going to go and do something bad."
4. 57	COUNSELOR	"You've just sort of shared with a small group of people how things went this weekend. How did it feel to share that with some people you know but other people who don't know you?" QUESTIONING to challenge individual feeling in context
4. 58	LIZ	"Um, it's kind of hard because you don't really know them, and so you don't know if they are going to go out and tell people and stuff. So . . ."
4. 59	COUNSELOR	"So that is sort of what you are wondering about in your mind after you've told people now. So it's sort of like a question with you, almost asking the group a question. 'I wonder if you guys are going to go out and say something.'" PARAPHRASING to acknowledge individual experience
4. 60	MARIA	"I think sometimes you feel kind of weird too because you don't know if they look at you differently now."
4. 61	COUNSELOR	"So it sounds like we have a second question out here now. In other words, are you going to tell someone and do you look at me differently now because I've shared that, you know, I have a problem at home?" PARAPHRASING to acknowledge individual experience
4. 62	KYLE	"That's why some people are afraid to share their feelings because then people might look at them different and have different opinions about them than what you want."
4. 63	COUNSELOR	"And taking that a step further, are you going to see Liz differently?" QUESTIONING to challenge individual experience
4. 64	KYLE	"I know her, but I don't talk to her much. I don't know her that well, but it doesn't make me think anything differently about her than I already did."

4. 65	COUNSELOR	"Amanda, I was just wanting to check in briefly with you, if maybe you could share with the group how are you feeling about being a member. I know that you have been listening, and I'm just wondering how's it going for you being a member here today?" QUESTIONING to challenge individual feeling with immediacy in context
4. 66	AMANDA	"Well, it's good to know that you can just kinda speak your mind and say what you're feeling and stuff and know that nobody else is going to say anything. But sometimes people aren't going to say anything because they kind of assume that other people are gonna go out and tell people what you said."
4. 67	COUNSELOR	"What I was going to do now is move into what we talked about last week, and that was getting at looking at the issue of anger, and anger is just one of many feelings. What I thought we could do, if it would work with the group, is just to look at and start naming some different kinds of feelings. We have a board up here, and we can write them down. I was wondering if there was a volunteer that would be willing to write down the feelings as members of the group contribute to naming off and calling out some different feelings." DIRECTING to challenge group feeling
4. 68	RACHEL	"I will."
4. 69	COUNSELOR	"OK, all right, all right."

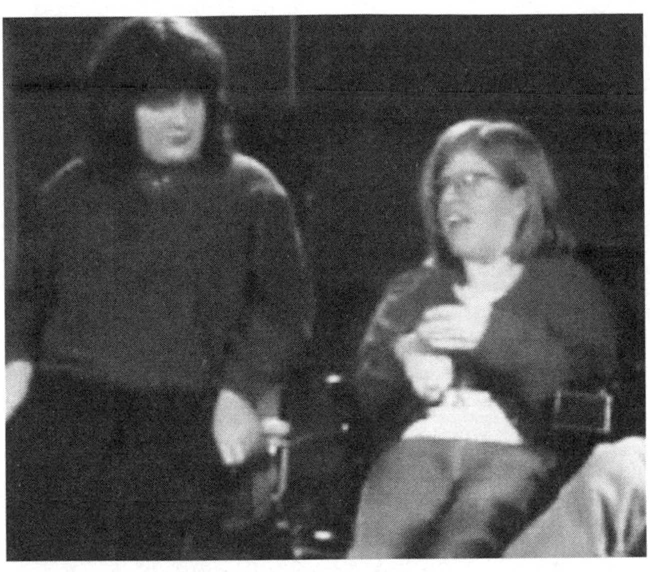

Transcript of Group 5/Adults

5. 1	COUNSELOR A	"It's always hard to know where a group's going to start . . . what it is that you want to talk about to begin with, and that's up to you." OPENING to acknowledge group experience
5. 2	CAROL	"I guess I would start by saying that I am kind of nervous about being in a group. And I have never been in one before. And I don't know how safe this group of people is to share things that are really personal to me. So . . . I would like to start just by being up front about that."
5. 3	COUNSELOR A	"Thank you, Carol. My hunch is that a lot of people here are nervous about that." PLAYING A HUNCH to challenge group feeling
5. 4	MATT	"That's probably why I'm being so quiet." (laughs)
5. 5	COUNSELOR A	"Can you say more about that?" CLARIFYING to explore individual behavior
5. 6	MATT	"Well, just trying to get a feel for things before I really start to say a lot about myself and, you know, some personal stuff. I kinda guess, waiting to see if it is a safe thing."
5. 7	COUNSELOR B	"Are other people feeling kinda the same, reticence in terms of, 'I don't know who these people are, and is it safe?'" QUESTIONING to challenge group feeling

5. 8	KEVIN	"For me, it isn't so much the fear of not knowing who everyone is . . . as much as it is how different we might be. If we'll have the same thoughts. Well, not necessarily the same thoughts, but if we'll be thinking along the same lines. That's sort of a concern for me."
5. 9	COUNSELOR A	"Wondering if you'll fit in?" PARAPHRASING to acknowledge individual thought *In question form*
5. 10	KEVIN	"Yeah, more or less."
5. 11	LOUISE	"I think I have a sort of strange concern when I sit here is that I am always worried that I'm gonna talk too much, that I'm gonna be the one that says stuff. So, I try to wait and see what everybody else, what everybody else says before I run over everybody or something."
5. 12	SHELLEY	"I kinda feel that same way, 'cause I know that I tend to talk a lot, so I try to hold back if I'm in a group so I don't take over."
5. 13	COUNSELOR B	"So, in some ways kinda the opposite concern, 'We're afraid we might not talk enough because we don't know who you are,' and you guys are afraid that, 'We'll go out there and dominate.'" PARAPHRASING to acknowledge subgroup behavior
5. 14	CAROL	"I know that with working and trying to go to school at the same time that I really don't feel that I have enough space for me. It seems like I'm running from class, to work, or some kind of other obligation in between. And I just don't have any time to think anymore and, and you know, I question whether or not I'm doing the right thing or if I'm overloading myself or . . . There's other times when I think that it is only another year and I can handle it but then I worry about whether or not I am short-changing myself."
5. 15	MATT	"The way I think about it when I find myself doing all that rushing around and not finding time for me and for . . . I wonder if I've got my priorities straight in what I'm doing and that's kinda bothersome because I think I do, but, but the way I've got my priorities right now it doesn't allow me a lot of time to do . . . to have fun and enjoy family time, so . . . that's kind of . . . I don't really know what to do with that."
5. 16	COUNSELOR A	"So you're both really busy. Your lives are busy and taken up with tasks? Is that what I'm hearing?" PARAPHRASING to acknowledge subgroup experience *In question form*

5. 17	CAROL	"Yeah. I mean for me it just seems like, you know, little things that normally wouldn't bother me, like, oh, I'm running 10 minutes late and I'm going to have to take the next bus. . . . It really throws me off, and that's not my personality usually, you know. I take things as they come and I don't sweat things like that, but now it's like 'Oh, 10 minutes late and the world's gonna come to an end!' And that's not every day, but it seems like I feel, that happens more often than it used to."
5. 18	LOUISE	"I think I identify too, with a lot of what you're saying in terms of you said something about it feeling like it's not really your personality. Because I feel like I'm doing a lot of things right now, I'm presenting myself as this person that's totally other than really how I have normally seen myself. Like I usually see myself as pretty solid and I think that my friends usually see me as pretty solid, and I feel like for the last 2 or 3 months everybody that I have come in contact with has seen this like, frazzled like, person that is totally late and has all this . . . you know, and missed, or forgot something to bring. I mean I just, I feel like I am just totally scattered when I come in contact with people and that they . . . I don't know if that's similar to how you mean by it being out of your personality, but that's how it feels like to me."
5. 19	CAROL	"Yeah, it feels like that to me, too, sometimes."
5. 20	COUNSELOR A	"Well, my hunch is there are people here who identify with that and people who don't. PLAYING A HUNCH to challenge subgroup experience
5. 21	AMY	"It's kinda true for me in some ways, when I'm busy. But, I kind of like to be busy, and I try to pack my day with more things and just keep things going at a really fast pace. And I think it's also because, I mean, I want it that way because I don't want to settle down. Just 'cause I don't want to stop and think about things. So, it's kind of like a blocking thing to keep it really, really busy."
5. 22	COUNSELOR A	"It's intentional?" QUESTIONING to explore individual behavior
5. 23	AMY	"Yeah."
5. 24	COUNSELOR A	"Not necessary or something that you have to be doing right now, but it's . . . " PARAPHRASING to acknowledge individual behavior
5. 25	AMY	"No. I'll find like little things. I mean, some of it can be procrastination, but a lot of it is just 'cause I don't want to be still."

5. 26	SHELLEY	"When I was listening to a lot of this stuff it wasn't necessarily, is not necessarily where I am at right now. But, if I try . . . I was kind of trying to think of where I am in relation to what a lot of people are saying and as far as . . . Like, for me right now my schedule . . . kind of like what you were saying, my schedule is really busy. But . . . but for me it's forced me . . . Like, right now, and I don't always do this, when I have a busy schedule. But for me it's forced me to be really organized. And I've found that I've been able to . . . like a lot of times . . . because I teach and I a lot of times will bring papers home to grade and that kind of stuff, and sometimes I get to a point where I feel that I am never off the job and it's really stressful. And lately it has been because I've been because I knew that like with the class that I am taking this quarter and stuff, I knew that I was going to be a lot busier than usual. I dropped a couple of commitments at work, some after-school stuff, and so I have been getting my work done there, and so I don't get home until later in the evening, but when I get home I don't have anything to do. I can just be there. So for me that part has been really nice lately. Because I feel like I'm, I don't know, it almost feels like my work is more compartmentalized, and even though I'm thinking about it and stuff . . . I love my job and all but I feel like it is more something I can leave at work and I'm not always dragging stuff home with me and doing it. So that part of it feels good right now. I guess I-Wei hasn't said much, either."
5. 27	I-WEI	"I'm just feeling really nervous. It makes me more nervous to see how comfortable you guys all look. So . . . I'm just trying to calm down."
5. 28	COUNSELOR A	"My hunch is some people don't feel as comfortable as they all look." PLAYING A HUNCH to challenge subgroup feeling
5. 29	LOUISE	"I can vouch for that."
5. 30	AMY	"I'm really good at that. I can give off this calm, cool, collected exterior, and inside I'm like, 'Oh no!' or something, you know? So . . ."
5. 31	COUNSELOR A	"Yeah. You feel nervous, too." EMPATHIZING to acknowledge individual feeling
5. 32	AMY	"A little bit, yeah."
5. 33	COUNSELOR A	"You feel nervous, too." EMPATHIZING to acknowledge individual feeling
5. 34	LOUISE	"Um-hmm. But it makes me more comfortable to talk, but that's my personality. It's that I'm a little more comfortable if I just talk."

5. 35	COUNSELOR A	"A strategy, kind of." PARAPHRASING to acknowledge individual behavior
5. 36	LOUISE	"I don't have to listen to my . . ." (laughs)
5. 37	COUNSELOR B	"So it seems like we all have a little bit of a discrepancy between kind of this outer image persona, smiling, laughing, nervous laughter, a lot, and how we are really feeling." NOTING A DESCREPANCY to challenge group behavior and feeling
5. 38	I-WEI	"It's basically hard for me to talk in front of so many people. But I'm trying to say something. I want to say something. I said that I want to take more risk than . . ."
5. 39	COUNSELOR A	"Yes." *Not a counseling response*
5. 40	KEVIN	"I have something that I would kind of throw out to the group, kind of see how other people are feeling. I don't really feel like I'm in control of my life right now. And I was just wondering what other people are thinking."
5. 41	COUNSELOR A	"You feel out of control." EMPATHIZING to acknowledge individual feeling
5. 42	KEVIN	"I do, yeah. I'm happy, you know, as I said before about some of the things I'm involved in, but I don't feel like I'm in control."
5. 43	COUNSELOR A	"And 'in control' or 'out of control' means . . . " QUESTIONING to challenge individual feeling
5. 44	KEVIN	". . . that things are going the way I want them to necessarily. I might be making choices that I might be happy with, but I'm not convinced that things have to be this way."
5. 45	COUNSELOR B	"But Kevin, isn't another way of saying that, 'How do I consistently make choices that put me in a situation where I feel out control?'" REFRAMING to challenge individual thought
5. 46	KEVIN	"Good point."
5. 47	CAROL	"What do you mean by 'consistently make choices'? I'm not sure what you mean by that because it seems Kevin's doing the best he can with a lot of stuff, and you know, it may not feel really good, but I'm sensing that you're probably doing the best you can."
5. 48	LOUISE	"I feel like now I'm more in control of my life than I've probably ever been, but I'm also more being controlled by all of the things that I've brought into my life that I . . . I don't know if that makes

		sense. But, like I have all of these things going on now, and so I'm in control because I'm able to organize all these things, but it also puts me in a position where I can be thrown easier by something new coming in because it's already so packed."
5. 49	COUNSELOR A	"I'm wondering since so many of you feel so out of control outside of the group if you're working hard to control the experience of the group now?" QUESTIONING to challenge subgroup behavior with immediacy in context
5. 50	AMY	"I don't really know if I can control the whole group. I mean I can just do what I can do. I mean, you know . . . I can't make people talk, and I can't make people be quiet, so I can't really control the group."
5. 51	COUNSELOR A	"Are you controlling yourself now?" QUESTIONING to challenge individual behavior with immediacy
5. 52	AMY	"Probably."
5. 53	COUNSELOR A	"Can you say more about that?" QUESTIONING to challenge individual experience
5. 54	AMY	"I don't know. I mean . . . But then I don't want to sound like, I don't know, it's kind of weird. I guess I don't want to say a whole lot yet 'cause I'm still trying to see where everybody is going to be in the group or who's or what the group is like, I guess, so in that sense I'm kind of controlling what I'm saying even though I am saying things in my head that I'm not saying them . . ."
5. 55	COUNSELOR B	"You're screening what you are saying." PARAPHRASING to acknowledge individual experience
5. 56	AMY	"Yeah."
5. 57	COUNSELOR A	"In a way to control what the group response might be to you or not, just let it go . . . " PLAYING A HUNCH to challenge individual behavior
5. 58	AMY	"I guess. Yeah, more as to keep myself in control. So maybe instead keeping the group in control, I'm keeping myself in control."
5. 59	COUNSELOR B	"In a way you control the group. Because you get to control, at least you think you control their responses, right? So if I don't let out too much then I don't know what I'd get back, but I can be sure of what I won't get back . . ." PLAYING A HUNCH to challenge individual behavior in context
5. 60	AMY	"That's true."

5. 61	COUNSELOR B	". . . I won't get back some judgment or rejection or 'Boy, am I weird.' So in a way . . ." *Continuation of 5.59*
5. 62	AMY	"Yeah."
5. 63	SHELLEY	"In a way, then, we're not really talking about a lot 'cause like when you say about being out of control, like I don't feel like I feel out of control outside of this group and so I don't know that I can necessarily relate with that. And I was sitting here . . . I guess I'm kinda controlling my experience in this group because I am kind of refraining from saying some of the things that I am thinking, but I really don't think that I'm . . . I don't want to say fitting in, but like in a way I kind of don't feel like I'm getting much out of this discussion in some ways and so, but I mean if we're not willing to talk about the stuff that is a little bit deeper, I don't mean to direct that at you, but I just mean in general, that we're not going to get anything out if it."
5. 64	COUNSELOR A	"And if you're not willing to talk about what's important, you're not going to get anything out of it." PARAPHRASING to acknowledge individual feeling
5. 65	SHELLEY	"Right. But I know another way, too. I kind of feel like I came in here with ideas of what I wanted to talk about and listening to this I feel more like, more together than I did when I came in here (laughs). So I don't know. So in some ways I feel kind of at a loss of what to say. But I don't necessarily feel like this is where I'm at."
5. 66	COUNSELOR B	"How are the people feeling right now for whom being out of control is an issue and is important?" QUESTIONING to challenge subgroup feeling with immediacy
5. 67	MATT	"I guess I'm feeling kind of frustrated by it because it is important to me and it appears like it's important to Kevin and other people, too. So I felt like it was something good, and it's not to say that you have to feel like it is something good, too, but I don't hear you coming up with anything else for the group to try and address, and so I feel like we've gotten off track of one thing that a lot of us are getting something out of, without going to another thing that people are getting something out of. It's kind of frustrating to me, especially since I was so engrossed in what we were talking about. That is coming from where I am."
5. 68	COUNSELOR A	"This has really fit for this part of the group. This was a theme that was very real, is very real." NOTING A THEME to acknowledge subgroup experience
5. 69	LOUISE	"But I think that even when we were talking about it I had a concern that . . . I had this sort of sense of 'OK, are we wasting some people's time, because this isn't their thing or what?' It feels like,

		it feels even like this has become more of a problem to me because I want to connect with everybody and I want us to have a common something so that everybody can feel like they're getting something or talking. . . ."
5. 70	MATT	"Well, if they're not going to talk, it's, I mean, then they're choosing to not do that. I mean . . ."
5. 71	LOUISE	"But that is how I feel in my life, too, like I'm responsible for everybody."
5. 72	SHELLEY	"Well, I guess that's why I was hesitant at first to say anything 'cause I didn't . . . 'cause obviously a lot people were connecting with that whole idea, but it wasn't . . . I don't know, it just is a response to my own questions. It is just not where I was at."
5. 73	COUNSELOR A	"How did it feel to have Matt say that he was frustrated with you?" QUESTIONING to challenge individual feeling
5. 74	SHELLEY	". . . It's fine. I can understand the frustration because I mean it seemed the majority of the group was talking about one thing, and I'm saying that I'm not really interested in that and . . . I don't know, maybe it means that I shouldn't be in this group. I don't know. It . . . I don't know. I guess it doesn't bother me that he's frustrated with it. I feel like . . . part of my concern was whether or not . . . I've kind of laid out all my options and had that laid out, and right now I am feeling like well, maybe I have the tools to make those decisions when they come and I really don't need to worry about that. I mean, I don't know. That sounded like I kind of, I was washing over the whole thing. But kind of the whole idea was that like the more I listen the more the more I feel like I've kind of got it together and I can probably deal with it and maybe I'm in a better position than I thought I was when I came into the group."
5. 75	AMY	"So listening to all of us makes you feel better about how you've got it all together?"
5. 76	SHELLEY	"Well, yeah."
5. 77	COUNSELOR A	"How does that make you feel?" QUESTIONING to challenge individual feeling
5. 78	AMY	"Very badly. I mean . . . I'm not that . . . I don't feel like my problems are that big. I mean it's not like I can't survive through the day. But I don't like being compared that, you know, listening to me, you have all these things put together now. I mean, unless I could go out and bottle it and make a whole bunch of money off of it, like, you know, 'Listen to me and you'll feel so much better about your life'" (laughs).

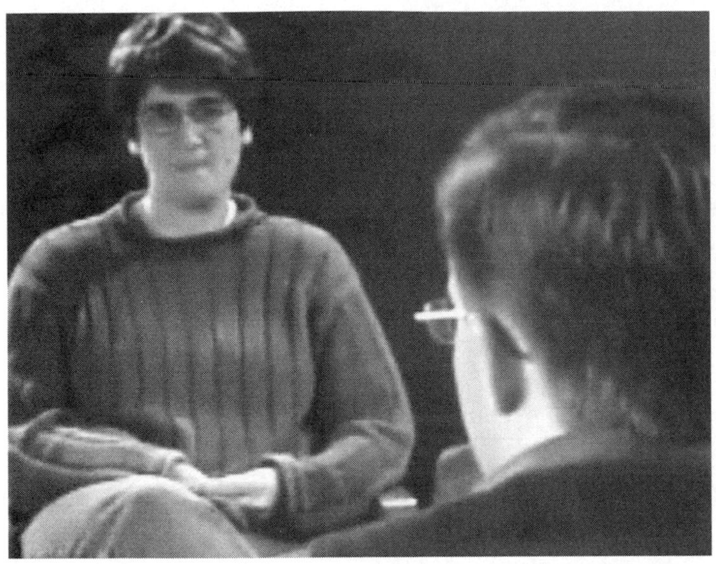

5. 79	MATT	"See, I have a different reaction then. You know, I am glad that you are getting something out of this, because what we were talking about before I was getting something out of. And it sounds like you actually were getting something out of this, despite what you said earlier that you weren't. And so . . ."
5. 80	SHELLEY	"That's true."
5. 81	COUNSELOR A	"It seems like the group is really wanting everybody to be able to get something out of this." PARAPHRASING to acknowledge group feeling
5. 82	KEVIN	"I do. I, you know, the thing for me is right when I came in, I didn't expect . . . and you might remember I said that I didn't know what other people were going to be thinking. You know, I really didn't expect that we were all going to think the same or feel the same or have the same concerns. So I mean I'm not surprised or offended or concerned, you know, that one of the group members doesn't, you know, have the same experiences going on right now. That's really OK with me. . . . I don't know, I just didn't expect that we were all going to have the same concerns, and I think anybody who feels like they, that he or she doesn't, can identify in his or her own way. Like, like, What's your name? I'm sorry."
5. 83	SHELLEY	"Shelley."
5. 84	KEVIN	"Like Shelley's doing, she's talking about what's going on for her right now. In her own way. Matt says she's getting something out of that."

5. 85	COUNSELOR A	"It makes sense to you that people don't have to be the same in order to . . ." PARAPHRASING to acknowledge individual feeling
5. 86	KEVIN	"Um-hmm. You know my reaction would be . . . I'm getting something from her about my situation. You know, I'm not judging myself based on what she said, but . . . just to hear her talk about her situation and think about my own, I'm getting her perspective, and that's helping me."
5. 87	COUNSELOR A	"How do you feel hearing that?" QUESTIONING to challenge individual feeling
5. 88	SHELLEY	". . . I guess in a way it feels . . . like, I don't know, I guess in a way I feel like maybe I could have like waited a little bit longer kind of to cut . . . I'm feeling like other people are feeling like they got cut off in this conversation about not being in of control and stuff. And . . . that maybe it would be a bit better to just kind of sit and wait until I've got a better idea about what I would like to talk about, but . . . I guess that is what I'm thinking right now."
5. 89	COUNSELOR A	"I wonder how it feels for people to see Shelley raise a different point of view and all of a sudden become the focus of the group." QUESTIONING to challenge group feeling in context
5. 90	CAROL	"I actually think that we learned something by listening to the dialogue here because I was kind of confused about how, when your life is so packed in with stuff, how you can regain control of that. Listening how, you know, Shelley's decisions about how to interact with the group, how there was space here to have some control, and even though I am making different choices in the group, I think that I can still try to apply some of those same things to things outside of the group when I start feeling busy."
5. 91	COUNSELOR A	"I wonder how it feels to people to see Shelley to be put on the hot seat." QUESTIONING to challenge group feeling
5. 92	KEVIN	"I have a thought. I'm a little uneasy about it . . . even though I'm on the other side of the issue's part, I don't really think she should be on the hot seat."
5. 93	LOUISE	"I think with that whole thing that there was one piece that I was uncomfortable with was when I thought Amy was uncomfortable with something Shelley said, and I could see myself having this sense of, 'No, no, no. Not here, too.' You know, I came here to get some sort of peace of . . . you know, and then it's like, wait, did I just and create a whole other thing that . . . "
5. 94	COUNSELOR A	"You feel like you created it." PARAPHRASING to challenge individual behavior

5. 95	LOUISE	"By being here, I created it being in my life. Not that I created any sort of difficulty between anybody else but that I invited another thing in my life that instead of being a piece of help it's going to be a piece of something else to sort out."
5. 96	COUNSELOR B	"So you invited conflict? That interpersonal, what you perceive to be interpersonal, conflict, and it's not what you need right now?" PARAPHRASING to acknowledge individual behavior
5. 97	LOUISE	"Yeah, I guess it just feels like that we are talking a lot about what's happening right here, right now with the group and everything, and so it feels like that's just a new thing that I have put in my, on my plate."
5. 98	I-WEI	"I don't know. But I was thinking that was very courageous of her."
5. 99	COUNSELOR A	"Can you tell her?" DIRECTING to challenge individual behavior *In question form*
5. 100	I-WEI	"I think that was very courageous of you. But I was also worried when I saw, when I heard what Matt said and Amy; I was really uncomfortable with that."
5. 101	COUNSELOR A	"How does it feel now?" QUESTIONING to challenge individual feeling with immediacy
5. 102	I-WEI	"I'm still wondering what Amy is thinking."
5. 103	COUNSELOR A	"Could you ask her?" DIRECTING to challenge individual behavior *In question form*
5. 104	I-WEI	"What are you feeling right now?"
5. 105	AMY	". . . I don't know, not great. 'Cause it's kind of like . . . I don't know. Like what I said, I should control what I say. . . . But then, another part of me is just feeling really uncomfortable just because everybody's kind of saying, 'Oh, Shelley just did this really good job, is really courageous in coming forward,' but when I said something that I really felt and I'm still having a problem with 'cause I don't even feel that it is really safe to talk, then people are saying that well, 'I feel uncomfortable with the conflict coming in, or I feel like, you know.' . . . So I'm feeling that I'm getting bad messages about what I said was wrong and what Shelley said was right, but I don't feel what Shelley did was right."
5. 106	COUNSELOR A	"Shelley is the good girl, and you are the bad girl." PARAPHRASING to challenge individual experience in context

5. 107	AMY	"Yeah."
5. 108	LOUISE	"That's weird because I don't feel like I felt uncomfortable that the conflict was created. I think I felt uncomfortable that I thought that you felt bad."
5. 109	AMY	"Oh, OK."
5. 110	LOUISE	"But I don't know if that, I mean, I don't know if that makes any difference to how you were feeling, but that's . . . like, I want everybody to feel good."
5. 111	AMY	"Yeah, it does."
5. 112	KEVIN	"I'm more in that position now. Because hearing Amy . . . you know, now she's now in the hot seat, and she's got to defend what she said. And so now I'll say to her what I said to Shelley. And that wasn't what I had in mind, you know. I didn't think that anybody would be put on the spot for anything that they said. You know, whether the group as a whole agreed or disagreed. You know, I thought it would be OK for everyone."
5. 113	I-WEI	"Amy, I just want you to know that I feel the same way as Louise. I felt uncomfortable just because I thought you were uncomfortable and Matt had a chance to comment on what he was thinking afterwards, but you did not get to say anything, so I was wondering."
5. 114	AMY	"Yeah . . . I'll be OK."
5. 115	COUNSELOR B	"So, seems like part of the issue that we're wrestling with is, can we be who we are, even if it disagrees with or challenges what other people might have said." PLAYING A HUNCH to challenge group experience
5. 116	MATT	"I feel like we're trying to put a good face on it. That's what I hear a lot of people doing, is trying to put people at ease. And say, like, 'What you did was OK' and 'We're happy you did that.'"
5. 117	COUNSELOR A	"How do you feel about that, Matt?" QUESTIONING to challenge individual feeling
5. 118	MATT	"Like, I wonder if it's really how people are feeling. I mean, I'm fine with people not agreeing that what I think is important is not important. I mean, you know, they don't have to think what I feel is important to me, and I know people aren't going to feel the same way about, but . . ."
5. 119	COUNSELOR A	"But you don't think everybody is not being honest about that?" QUESTIONING to challenge individual thought *In question form*
5. 120	MATT	"Yeah, yeah."

5. 121	COUNSELOR A	"Who do you think is not being honest?" QUESTIONING to challenge individual thought
5. 122	MATT	"Huh, probably all of us. I know I'm not being totally honest."
5. 123	COUNSELOR A	"If you were totally honest, what would you say now?" QUESTIONING to challenge individual thought with immediacy
5. 124	MATT	"I feel like we're just going around and around about something that really wasn't that big of a deal, and we should get past it. And people aren't getting past it."
5. 125	COUNSELOR A	"Feel frustrated?" EMPATHIZING to acknowledge individual feeling
5. 126	MATT	"Yeah. Yeah."
5. 127	LOUISE	"I guess I feel like if we just get past it . . ."
5. 128	MATT	"I feel like I'm in Shelley's position earlier, actually (laughs). I feel like it's a waste of time what we've been doing for the last, I don't know how long, but and maybe that's just because I was really into what we were doing before we shifted gears, and I'm just not able to make that transition, but I feel like this is a waste of time. I'll say it again."
5. 129	COUNSELOR A	"You feel like your time is being wasted." EMPATHIZING to acknowledge individual feeling
5. 130	MATT	"Yeah. Yeah."
5. 131	I-WEI	"I feel uncomfortable about what he said, because I think he doesn't know who's being honest and who's not. Maybe he's not being totally honest, but he doesn't know if we're being dishonest."
5. 132	COUNSELOR A	"Would you talk to . . ." DIRECTING to challenge individual behavior
5. 133	I-WEI	"And that's how I feel. I think you're making a judgment. And I think that by saying that . . . Actually, that's taking a risk. It's hard for me to say that, but . . . I think earlier I was concerned about Amy because I don't want us to just keep going, and then she didn't get to say what she has to say and feeling uncomfortable about left out. That's why I made that comment. I kind of feel like you were directing that comment toward me."
5. 134	MATT	"About my comment about feeling like it was . . ."
5. 135	I-WEI	"About trying to make people feel better and making sure that . . ."
5. 136	MATT	"I wasn't directing it solely at you. I mean, I was directing it at Louise, Kevin, other people, too."

5. 137	I-WEI	"But the truth is you don't know what we're feeling."
5. 138	MATT	"Right."
5. 139	COUNSELOR A	"It strikes me this is like the theme, Matt, of having those things that you want to accomplish and having other people that have other agendas, sort of. Sort of like here that, that, theme that we were talking about in the life sort of comes here in the group, too." NOTING A THEME to challenge individual experience in context
5. 140	MATT	"I'm trying to be as honest as I can about how I'm feeling, so I would assume that other people would do the same thing, and that is an assumption and a judgment. So before, I felt safe enough to share that and, you know, went out a little bit beyond where I was really comfortable with and said that, knowing that people were probably going to react to it. I was kind of hoping for that kind that people were going to get involved."
5. 141	SHELLEY	"I think that kind of goes along with what Louise was saying, too, about how, even though we're not going to agree about the idea of it, still feeling safe to talk about things. And when I had said what I had said it obviously upset you, and that wasn't my intention, but regardless, it still upset you. But I would hope that even if we say things that are upsetting, kind of like what you are saying right now, if it is upsetting to someone else, that wouldn't mean that it would close off conversation, that like you or I could disagree, or any of us could disagree and still be able to talk and be able to say openly what we are thinking and . . ."
5. 142	COUNSELOR A	"I see heads nodding a little bit." GIVING FEEDBACK to acknowledge group behavior
5. 143	CAROL	"I'm glad we're listening to each other. . . . I started to feel like, you know, for a little bit, that we were more concerned about what we were going to say rather than listening to other people in the group. I think that not everybody is going to say things that are the same for me. That's OK, but sometimes I can still learn from it, and even if it's not the same. Like you, what I was saying before about Shelley, listening to her and how she was able to control herself in the group, was really helpful for me."
5. 144	COUNSELOR A	"You identify with that?" QUESTIONING to challenge individual experience
5. 145	CAROL	"Yeah, well, I didn't at first because I was struggling with how I could have control in my life, and this is kind of an example of choices. And that was something that had been talked about earlier that I wasn't quite understanding, and so this kind of helped me to see where the choice was. And that was helpful, so in that case it was helpful for me to listen and not necessarily talk."

5. 146	COUNSELOR B	"I wonder if the same reticence we had about making the choices to disagree in here might also be part of the choices we make that make us end up with schedules we really don't want." NOTING A CONNECTION to challenge group thought and behavior in context
5. 147	COUNSELOR A	"Anyone have something that we want to say?" CLOSING to acknowledge group experience *In question form*
5. 148	LOUISE	"I just found in the last like, I think, ten minutes probably that my energy level just went, hit the floor, because I think I realized that this is going to be work, and I didn't think I was going to be working. Yeah. So it is sort of a resetting of my approach or my or the way that I'm thinking about this and the way that I need to be when I'm here in terms of my . . ."
5. 149	COUNSELOR A	"It's going to be work." PARAPHRASING to acknowledge individual experience
5. 150	LOUISE	"Yeah, in terms of maybe I need to go down a little bit deeper. Yeah, that's it. That's what I have."

Follow-up of Group Clients

Four months after the completion of the taping of the group video, clients were contacted by phone and asked to respond to the following three questions:

1. What was the most meaningful thing that you heard in the group session?
2. Who said it?
3. Do you have any other feedback about the group experience?

Out of the 38 total client participants, 23 individuals were reached and responded to the three questions listed above. Below are the direct quotes of each client contacted.

Group 1/Women

Sue:

1. An African American and another woman in the group both talked about being treated differently because of circumstances beyond their control.
2. Clients.
3. The group experience was different than expected. I was surprised at the powerful emotions that emerged.

Barbara:

1. "It sounds like you are angry with me."
2. Counselor.
3. Group process is a wonderful process. After 3 years, I learned a lot about the people around me.

Dorothy:

1. Others sharing similar experience to my own.
2. Clients.
3. The experience was wonderful. It was interesting to go from opening to closing within a few hours. I had a great time. The technical staff disappeared into the background nicely. The group leader was appropriate and professional. Role-playing experience in classes was a good preparation for the experience.

Lynn:

1. When I heard others say that my feelings were OK to have.
2. Clients.
3. It was amazing how quickly people became open and shared in spite of the lighting and technical crew.

Vee:

1. When one of the group members acknowledged her true feelings about not participating in the group and needing attention all the time.
2. Clients.
3. We got into genuine processing in somewhat artificial circumstances.

Group 2/Boys

Rick:

1. That some of the people don't have ways to get their anger out and they must go to the weight room and lift.
2. Client.
3. It was fun. And interesting to hear what other people had to say—especially my brother, because I never heard him talk that much.

Wallace:

1. Everybody talking about their backgrounds. Even though I hang out with those guys, it was great to hear what they've been through. It's great to know somebody else out there knows what I've gone through. Other people can understand where I'm coming from.
2. Clients.
3. It was fun to hear others talk and get together. That's basically it.

Mitchell:

1. People expressing their thoughts on life. Reasons they do stuff. Like one of the guys said the reason he does sports harder and stuff.
2. Clients.
3. It helped me understand where people are coming from. Like one of the guys I live with—he never said anything like that before. It helped me understand why people do the things they do.

James:

1. I do not know.
2. I don't know.
3. I expressed my opinions, my view and how it related to other people.

Eric:

1. That it was a cool group. It was cool to be able to talk about stuff without people making fun of you.
2. Clients.
3. I don't know.

Group 3/Graduates

Amy:

1. I don't remember anything specifically that was said. It has been too long ago. Most of the clients talked about being frustrated with the graduate program and wanted to be done. One client didn't feel that way. That is all I remember about it.
2. Clients.
3. It was all pretty interesting.

Aaron:

1. "I don't think it matters what the group counselors think."
2. A client, Amy, made the comment.
3. I liked discussing why it's so hard to get to know people while in this program. I wish we had time to process that more.

Kara:

1. I can't remember exactly but there were comments about member anxiety about where they were at in the program. They were questioning what they wanted to do. That was the most important issue. I was feeling similar thoughts and concluded I'm not alone.
2. The clients.
3. I was amazed at the fact that despite the microphones and lights, the group process was not interrupted.

Darren:

1. Clients talked about their stress and fatigue while being in the graduate program. It affects us all. People are pushed to the limit. Maybe depression is the result.
2. Clients.
3. I thought the co-facilitators did a good job.

Nicole:

1. I don't remember anything meaningful.
2. I don't know.
3. I felt like I didn't fit into the group. I'm too early in the program. My situation wasn't the same as others. Many talked about their internship. Maybe I was in the wrong group.

Group 4/Students

Rachel:

1. I remember "SODA." It stands for stop, options, decision, and act.
2. Taught by the counselor.
3. It was nice being able to talk to someone about this stuff.

Amanda:

1. It was too long ago. I can't remember anything.
2. I don't know.
3. I hope what we talked about helps someone. We talked about real life stuff.

Kyle:

1. I can't remember anything. It was so long ago.
2. I don't know.
3. I liked doing the group. I don't mind talking about how I feel.

Group 5/Adults

Shelley:

1. What stands out is the discussion of people trying to make sure their needs got met, and then there was conflict.
2. Clients.
3. It was interesting. I liked the group members. I would have enjoyed being in a long-term group with them. I liked that conflict was dealt with right away when it came up. That was a new experience for me.

Louise:

1. I remember what I said. I talked about feeling scattered.
2. Client.
3. At the beginning of the group, it felt like we were processing. Then we were cut off. I was hoping for more.

Matt:

1. Someone was confrontive to me, brought the group to a new level and we could then talk about our true feelings.
2. Client.
3. I had more experience in group process than the other members. I had already finished the program, and I led groups myself. I was in a different place and so took on a leadership role. Maybe I wouldn't have if there had been other members.

Amy:

1. The comment I remember most irritated me: "I don't want to be around sick people."
2. Client.
3. I liked being a part of the group. We went through all the stages in just one session.

Kevin:

1. What I remember most is that we could all experience something different, and it was OK. We didn't all have to agree. We could have a different focus.
2. Clients.
3. I thought it would be a certain kind of group. I was prepared for a group on being a graduate student. It was hard to switch gears. I wish I had known what kind of group I was participating in beforehand.

TABLE 1 COMPARING *BASIC COUNSELING RESPONSES IN GROUPS* TO RESPONSES/SKILLS OF OTHER MODELS

	Basis Counseling Responses in Groups	COREY *Theory and Practice of Group Counseling (5th Edition)*	JACOBS, MASSON, HARVILL *Group Counseling Skills and Strategies*	IVEY, PEDERSON, IVEY *Intentional Group Counseling: A Microskills Approach*	REID *Social Work Practice with Groups*
R E S P O N S E	OPENING OR CLOSING	Opening and closing Terminating			Getting started Closing the initial session, Termination
	ATTENDING	Active listening	Active listening Scanning for nonverbal clues	Attending Behavior	Active listening Scanning
	EMPATHIZING	Reflecting feelings Empathizing	Reflection	Reflection feeling Empathizing	Empathizing
	PARAPHRASING	Restating Summarizing	Summarizing Reflection	Paraphrasing Summarization	Summarizing Partializing
	GIVING FEEDBACK	Giving feedback	Feedback Influencing	Feedback	Giving feedback
	CLARIFYING	Clarifying	Clarification	Encouraging and restatement	Concreteness
	DIRECTING	Blocking, Facilitating, Initiating	Drawing out members Cutting off members	Leading, Pacing Structuring Strategies	Guiding interaction
	QUESTIONING	Questioning	Questioning	Open and closed questioning Eliciting and reflecting Meaning	Perception checks
	NOTING A CONNECTION	Linking		Interpretation	Synthesizing

RESPONSE	NOTING A THEME	Linking		Interpretation	
	NOTING A DISCREPANCY	Interpreting Confronting		Interpretation Confronting	Confronting discrepancies
	REFRAMING	Suggesting		Reframing	Reframing
	PLAYING A HUNCH	Interpreting		Interpretation	Confronting
	ALLOWING SILENCE				
	SELF-DISCLOSING	Self-disclosure	Self-disclosure	Self-disclosure	Self-disclosure
INTENT	ACKNOWLEDGE			Intentionality	
	EXPLORE			Intentionality	
	CHALLENGE			Intentionality	
FOCUS	INDIVIDUAL/SUBGROUP/ GROUP EXPERIENCE		Focus	Focusing group, subgroup, individual	Group or individual focus
	INDIVIDUAL/SUBGROUP/ GROUP FEELING		Focus	Focusing group, subgroup, individual	
	INDIVIDUAL/SUBGROUP/ GROUP THOUGHT		Focus	Focusing group, subgroup, individual	
	INDIVIDUAL/SUBGROUP/ GROUP BEHAVIOR		Focus	Focusing group, subgroup, individual	
	CONTEXT/IMMEDIACY	Here and now	Focus	Focusing here and now	Thinking in the here and now

Figure 1 RESPONSES

OPENING OR CLOSING	ATTENDING	EMPATHIZING
PARAPHRASING	GIVING FEEDBACK	QUESTIONING
CLARIFYING	DIRECTING	PLAYING A HUNCH
NOTING A THEME	NOTING A DISCREPANCY	NOTING A CONNECTION
REFRAMING	ALLOWING SILENCE	SELF-DISCLOSING

Figure 2 Intents

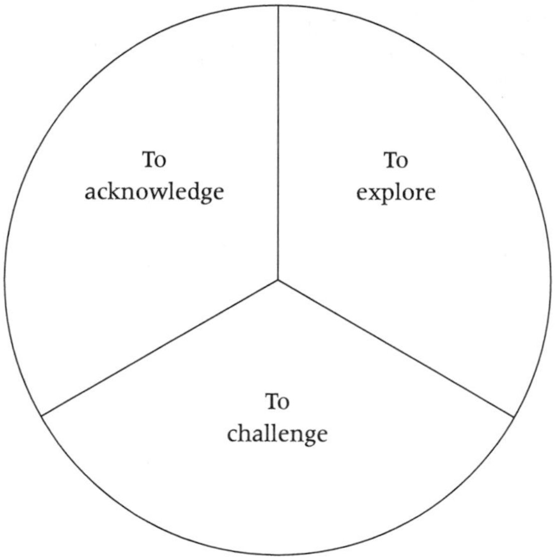

To acknowledge

To explore

To challenge

Figure 3 Group Focus

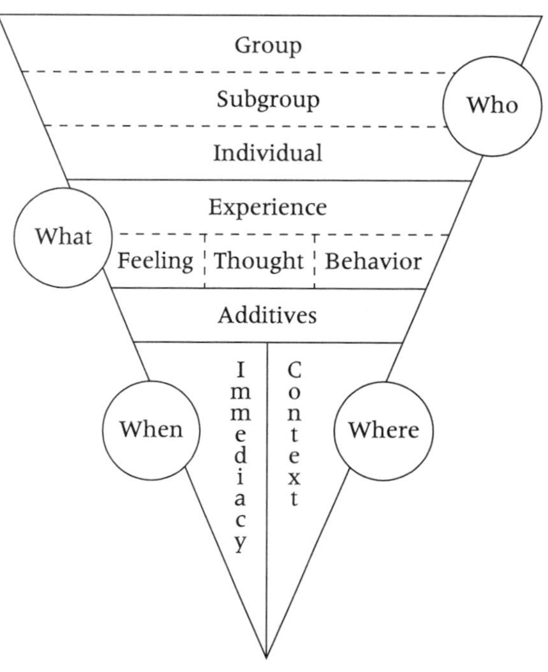

APPENDIX B

Group Counseling Bibliography

Bates, M., Johnson, C. D., & Blaker, K. E. (1982). *Group leadership: A manual for group counseling leaders.* Denver, CO: Love Publishing.

Berg, R. C., Landreth, G. G., & Fall, K. A. (1998). *Group counseling: Concepts and procedures* (3rd ed.). Philadelphia: Taylor and Francis.

Brantley, L. S., Brantley, P. S., & Baer-Barkley, K. (1996). Transforming acting-out behavior: A group counseling program for inner-city elementary school pupils. *Elementary School Guidance and Counseling, 31 (2),* pp. 96–105.

Capuzzi, D., & Gross, D. R. (1998). *Introduction to group counseling* (2nd ed.). Denver, CO: Love Publishing.

Capuzzi, D., & Gross, D. R. (1998). *Student handbook for introduction to group counseling* (2nd ed.). Denver, CO: Love Publishing.

Carroll, M., Bates, M., & Johnson, C. (1997). *Group leadership: Strategies for group counseling leaders* (3rd ed.). Denver, CO: Love Publishing.

Corey, G. (2000). *Student manual for theory and practice of group counseling* (5th ed.). Pacific Grove, CA: Brooks/Cole.

Corey, G., Corey, M. S., Callanan, P., & Russell, J. M. (1992). *Group techniques* (2nd ed.). Pacific Grove, CA: Brooks/Cole.

Corey, M. S., and Corey, G., (1997). *Groups: process and practice* (5th ed.). Pacific Grove, CA Brooks/Cole.

Donigan, J., & Malnati, R. (1987). *Critical incidents in group therapy.* Monterey, CA: Brooks/Cole.

Donigan, J., & Malnati, R. (1997). *Systemic group therapy: A triadic model.* Pacific Grove, CA: Brooks/Cole.

Forsyth, D. R. (1983). *An approach to group dynamics.* Monterey, CA: Brooks/Cole.

Gazda, G. M. (1978). *Group counseling: A developmental approach* (2nd ed.). Boston: Allyn and Bacon.

Goldberg, C. (1970). *Encounter: Groups sensitivity training experience.* New York: Science House.

Johnson, D. W., & Johnson, F. P. (1997). *Joining together: Group therapy and group skills* (6th ed.). Boston: Allyn and Bacon.

Kizner, L. R., & Kizner, S. R. (1999). Small group counseling with adopted children. *Professional School Counseling, 2(3),* pp. 226–229.

Lacoursiere, R. B. (1980). *The life cycle of groups: Group developmental stage theory.* New York: Human Sciences Press.

Lieberman, M. A., Yalom, I. D., & Miles, M. B. (1973). *Encounter groups: First facts.* New York: Basic Books.

McManus, R., & Jennings, G. (eds.) (1996). *Structured exercises for promoting family and group strengths: A handbook for group leaders, trainers, educators, counselors, and therapists.* New York: Haworth Press.

Merritt, R. E., Jr., & Walley, D. D. (1977). *The group leader's handbook: Resource, techniques, and survival skills.* Champaign, IL: Research Press.

Naar, R. (1982). *A primer of group psychotherapy.* New York: Human Sciences Press.

Napier, R. W., & Gershenfeld, M. K. (1993). *Groups: Theory and experience* (5th ed.). Boston: Houghton Mifflin.

Ohlsen, M. M., Horne, A. M., & Lawe, C. F. (1988). *Group counseling* (3rd ed.). New York: Holt, Rinehart and Winston.

Ormont, L. R. (1992). *The group therapy experience: From theory to practice.* New York: St. Martins Press.

Riddle, J., Bergin, J. J., & Douzenis, C. (1997). Effects of group counseling on the self-concept of children of alcoholics. *Elementary School Guidance and Counseling, 31(3),* pp. 192–203.

Schmuck, R. A., & Schmuck, P. A. (1997). *Group processes in the classroom* (7th ed.). Madison, WI: Brown and Benchmark.

Shaffer, J. B. P., & Galinsky, M. D. (1989). *Models of group therapy* (2nd ed.). Englewood Cliffs, NJ: Prentice-Hall.

Shaw, M. E. (1981). *Group dynamics: The psychology of small group behavior* (3rd ed.). New York: McGraw-Hill.

Soloman, L. N., & Berzon, B. (eds.) (1972). *New perspectives on encounter groups.* San Francisco: Jossey-Bass.

Weiner, M. F. (1984). *Techniques of group psychotherapy.* Washington, DC: American Psychiatric Press.

Yalom, I. D. (1983). *Inpatient group psychotherapy.* New York: Basic Books.

Specialized Bibliography

Ethics

Berg, R. C., Landreth, G. L., & Fall, K. A. (1998). Holistic leadership training. *Group counseling: Concepts and procedures* (3rd ed.) (pp. 63–136). Philadelphia: Taylor & Francis.

Carroll, M., Bates, M., & Johnson, C. (1997). Common unethical behaviors. *Group leadership: Strategies for group counseling leaders* (3rd ed.) (pp. 299–307). Denver, CO: Love Publishing.

Corey, G. (2000). Ethical and professional issues in group practice. *Theory and practice of group counseling* (5th ed.) (pp. 63–84). Pacific Grove, CA: Brooks/Cole.

Corey, G., Corey, M. S., Callanan, P., & Russell, J. M. (1992). Ethical issues in using group techniques. *Group techniques* (2nd ed.) (pp. 17–32). Pacific Grove, CA: Brooks/Cole.

Corey, M. S., & Corey, G. (1997). Ethical and legal issues in group counseling. *Groups: Process and practice* (5th ed.) (pp. 25–58). Pacific Grove, CA: Brooks/Cole.

Forester-Miller, H. (1998). Group counseling: Ethical considerations. D. Capuzzi, & D. R. Gross (Eds.). *Introduction to group counseling* (2nd ed.) (pp. 159–178). Denver, CO: Love Publishing.

Gladding, S. T. (1999). Ethical and legal aspects of group work. *Group work: A counseling specialty* (3rd ed.) (pp. 213–237). Upper Saddle River, NJ: Prentice–Hall.

Johnson, D. W., & Johnson, F. P. (1997). Ethics of experiential learning. *Joining together: Group theory and group skills* (6th ed.) (pp. 66–69). Boston: Allyn and Bacon.

Weiner, M. F. (1984). Ethical and legal issues. *Techniques of group psychotherapy* (pp. 231–239). Washington, DC: American Psychiatric Press.

Diversity

Arciniega, M., & Newlon, B. J. (1998). Multicultural group counseling: Cross-cultural considerations. D. Capuzzi, & D. R. Gross (Eds.). *Introduction to group counseling* (2nd ed.) (pp. 181–202). Denver, CO: Love Publishing.

Berg, R. C., Landreth, G. L., & Fall, K. A. (1998). Group counseling with specific populations. *Group counseling: Concepts and procedures* (3rd ed.) (pp. 361–397). Philadelphia: Taylor & Francis.

Clark, J., & Blanchard, M. (1998). Group Counseling for people with addictions. D. Capuzzi, & D. R. Gross (Eds.). *Introduction to group counseling* (2nd ed.) (pp. 279–300). Denver, CO: Love Publishing.

Corey, G. (2000). Applying Behavior Therapy with multicultural populations. *Theory and practice of group counseling* (5th ed.) (pp. 455–465). Pacific Grove, CA: Brooks/Cole.

Corey, G. (2000). Applying Psychodrama with multicultural populations. *Theory and practice of group counseling* (5th ed.) (pp. 455–465). Pacific Grove, CA: Brooks/Cole.

Corey, G. (2000). Applying Rational Emotive Behavior Therapy with multicultural populations. *Theory and practice of group counseling* (5th ed.) (pp. 455–465). Pacific Grove, CA: Brooks/Cole.

Corey, G. (2000). Applying Reality Therapy with multicultural populations. *Theory and practice of group counseling* (5th ed.) (pp. 455–465). Pacific Grove, CA: Brooks/Cole.

Corey, G. (2000). Applying TA with multicultural populations. *Theory and practice of group counseling* (4th ed.) (pp. 455–465). Pacific Grove, CA: Brooks/Cole.

Corey, G. (2000). Applying the Adlerian approach with multicultural populations. *Theory and practice of group counseling* (5th ed.) (pp. 455–465). Pacific Grove, CA: Brooks/Cole.

Corey, G. (2000). Applying the Adlerian approach with multicultural populations. *Theory and practice of group counseling* (5th ed.) (pp. 455–465). Pacific Grove, CA: Brooks/Cole.

Corey, G. (2000). Applying the Existential approach with multicultural populations. *Theory and practice of group counseling* (5th ed.) (pp. 455–465). Pacific Grove, CA: Brooks/Cole.

Corey, G. (2000). Applying the Gestalt Therapy with multicultural populations. *Theory and practice of group counseling* (5th ed.) (pp. 455–465). Pacific Grove, CA: Brooks/Cole.

Corey, G. (2000). Applying the Person-Centered approach with multicultural populations. *Theory and practice of group counseling* (5th ed.) (pp. 455–465). Pacific Grove, CA: Brooks/Cole.

Corey, G. (2000). Group work in a multicultural context: Various perspectives. *Theory and practice of group counseling* (5th ed.) (pp. 455–465). Pacific Grove, CA: Brooks/Cole.

Corey, G., Corey, M. S., Callanan, P., & Russell, J. M. (1992). Choosing techniques for various types of groups. *Group techniques* (2nd ed.) (pp. 5–10). Pacific Grove, CA: Brooks/Cole.

Corey, M. S., & Corey, G. (1997). A multicultural perspective on group work. *Groups: Process and practice* (5th ed.) (pp. 14–17). Pacific Grove, CA: Brooks/Cole.

Corey, M. S., & Corey, G. (1997). Groups for adolescents. *Groups: Process and practice* (5th ed.) (pp. 321–358). Pacific Grove, CA: Brooks/Cole.

Corey, M. S., & Corey, G. (1997). Groups for adults. *Groups: Process and practice* (5th ed.) (pp. 359–405). Pacific Grove, CA: Brooks/Cole.

Corey, M. S., & Corey, G. (1997). Groups for children. *Groups: Process and practice* (5th ed.) (pp. 295–320). Pacific Grove, CA: Brooks/Cole.

Corey, M. S., & Corey, G. (1997). Groups for the elderly. *Groups: Process and practice* (5th ed.) (pp. 406–443). Pacific Grove, CA: Brooks/Cole.

Corey, M. S., & Corey, G. (1997). Multicultural awareness in group practice. *Groups: Process and practice* (5th ed.) (pp. 40–42). Pacific Grove, CA: Brooks/Cole.

Frank, M. L. B. (1998) Group counseling for individuals with eating disorders. D. Capuzzi, & D. R. Gross (Eds.). *Introduction to group counseling* (2nd ed.) (pp. 304–329). Denver, CO: Love Publishing.

Gladding, S. T. (1999). Group work with culturally diverse populations. *Group work: A counseling specialty* (3rd ed.) (pp. 195–211). Upper Saddle River, NJ: Prentice-Hall.

Gladding, S. T. (1999). Groups for adolescents. *Group work: A counseling specialty* (3rd ed.) (pp. 263–287). Upper Saddle River, NJ: Prentice-Hall.

Gladding, S. T. (1999). Groups for adults. *Group work: A counseling specialty* (3rd ed.) (pp. 289–319). Upper Saddle River, NJ: Prentice-Hall.

Gladding, S. T. (1999). Groups for children. *Group work: A counseling specialty* (3rd ed.) (pp. 239–261). Upper Saddle River, NJ: Prentice-Hall.

Gladding, S. T. (1999). Groups for the elderly. *Group work: A counseling specialty* (3rd ed.) (pp. 321–337). Upper Saddle River, NJ: Prentice-Hall.

Gladding, S. T. (1999). Influencing group dynamics: Preplanning. *Group work: A counseling specialty* (3rd ed.) (51–52). Upper Saddle River, NJ: Prentice-Hall.

House, R. M., & Tyler, V. (1998). Group counseling with gay, lesbian and bisexual clients. D. Capuzzi, & D. R. Gross (Eds.). *Introduction to group counseling* (2nd ed.) (pp. 359–388). Denver, CO: Love Publishing.

Johnson, D. W., & Johnson, F. P. (1997). Cross-ethnic conflict. *Joining together: Group theory and group skills* (6th ed.) (pp. 390–393). Boston: Allyn and Bacon.

Johnson, D. W., & Johnson, F. P. (1997). Dealing with diversity. *Joining together: Group theory and group skills* (6th ed.) (pp. 443–465. Boston: Allyn and Bacon.

Livneh, H. & Pullo, R. E. (1998). Group counseling for people with physical disabilities. D. Capuzzi, & D. R. Gross (Eds.). *Introduction to group counseling* (2nd ed.) (pp. 331–358). Denver, CO: Love Publishing.

Morganett, R. S. (1990). Guidelines for group success. *Skills for life: Group counseling activities for young adolescents* (pp. 7–10). Champaign, IL: Research Press.

Schmuck, R. A., Schmuck, P. A. (1997). Social basis of influence: Gender, race, and ethnicity. *Group processes in the classroom* (7th ed.) (pp. 68–70). Madison, WI: Brown & Benchmark.

Sherwood-Hawes, A. (1998). Group counseling for issues related to suicide. D. Capuzzi, & D. R. Gross (Eds.). *Introduction to group counseling* (2nd ed.) (pp. 415–444). Denver, CO: Love Publishing.

Thomas, M.C., & Martin, V. (1998). Group counseling with the elderly and their caregivers. D. Capuzzi, & D. R. Gross (Eds.). *Introduction to group counseling* (2nd ed.) (pp. 389–413). Denver, CO: Love Publishing.

Group Development

Berg, R. C., Landreth, G. L., & Fall, K. A. (1998). Initiating a counseling group. *Group counseling: Concepts and procedures* (3rd ed.) (pp. 157–208). Philadelphia: Taylor & Francis.

Berg, R. C., Landreth, G. L., & Fall, K. A. (1998). Maintaining a group: Process and development. *Group counseling: Concepts and procedures* (3rd ed.) (pp. 279–296). Philadelphia: Taylor & Francis.

Capuzzi, D. & Gross, D. R. (1998). Facilitating group stages. *Introduction to group counseling* (2nd ed.) (pp. 55–67). Denver, CO: Love Publishing.

Carroll, M., Bates, M., & Johnson, C. (1997). How people change in groups. *Group leadership: Strategies for group counseling leaders* (3rd ed.) (pp. 49–83). Denver, CO: Love Publishing.

Corey, G. (2000). Early stages of the development of a group. *Theory and practice of group counseling* (5th ed.) (pp. 87–113). Pacific Grove, CA: Brooks/Cole.

Corey, G. (2000). Person-Centered group process. *Theory and practice of group counseling* (5th ed.) (pp. 274–302). Pacific Grove, CA: Brooks/Cole.

Corey, G. (2000). Phases of the Adlerian group. *Theory and practice of group counseling* (5th ed.) (pp. 187–211). Pacific Grove, CA: Brooks/Cole.

Corey, G. (2000). Stages of a Behavior-Therapy group. *Theory and practice of group counseling* (5th ed.) (pp. 361–392). Pacific Grove, CA: Brooks/Cole.

Corey, G. (2000). The Gouldings' redecisional approach to groups. *Theory and practice of group counseling* (5th ed.) (pp. 338–359). Pacific Grove, CA: Brooks/Cole.

Corey, G., Corey, M. S., Callanan, P., & Russell, J. M. (1992). Characteristics of the initial stage. *Group techniques* (2nd ed.) (pp. 59–60). Pacific Grove, CA: Brooks/Cole.

Corey, G., Corey, M. S., Callanan, P., & Russell, J. M. (1992). Characteristics of the transition stage. *Group techniques* (2nd ed.) (pp. 81). Pacific Grove, CA: Brooks/Cole.

Corey, G., Corey, M. S., Callanan, P., & Russell, J. M. (1992). Characteristics of the working stage. *Group techniques* (2nd ed.) (pp. 115–119). Pacific Grove, CA: Brooks/Cole.

Corey, M. S., & Corey, G. (1997). Ending a group. *Groups: Process and practice* (5th ed.) (263–292). Pacific Grove, CA: Brooks/Cole.

Corey, M. S., & Corey, G. (1997). Group stages: process and development. *Groups: Process and practice* (5th ed.) (pp. 103–292). Pacific Grove, CA: Brooks/Cole.

Corey, M. S., & Corey, G. (1997). Initial stage of a group. *Groups: Process and practice* (5th ed.) (pp. 134–173). Pacific Grove, CA: Brooks/Cole.

Corey, M. S., & Corey, G. (1997). Transition stage of a group. *Groups: Process and practice* (5th ed.) (pp. 174–220). Pacific Grove, CA: Brooks/Cole.

Corey, M. S., & Corey, G. (1997). Working stage of a group. *Groups: Process and practice* (5th ed.) (pp. 221–262). Pacific Grove, CA: Brooks/Cole.

Donigan, J., & Malnati, R. (1997). Group stages. *Systemic group therapy: A triadic model* (pp. 53–80). Pacific Grove, CA: Brooks/Cole.

Donigan, J., & Malnati, R. (1997). Stages. *Systemic group therapy: A triadic model* (pp. 40–43). Pacific Grove, CA: Brooks/Cole.

Gladding, S. T. (1999). Beginning a group. *Group work: A counseling specialty* (3rd ed.) (pp. 103–126). Upper Saddle River, NJ: Prentice-Hall.

Gladding, S. T. (1999). Termination of a group. *Group work: A counseling specialty* (3rd ed.) (pp. 171–194). Upper Saddle River, NJ: Prentice-Hall.

Gladding, S. T. (1999). The transition period in a group: Norming and storming. *Group work: A counseling specialty* (3rd ed.) (pp. 127–148). Upper Saddle River, NJ: Prentice-Hall.

Gladding, S. T. (1999). The working stage in a group: Performing. *Group work: A counseling specialty* (3rd ed.) (pp. 149–170). Upper Saddle River, NJ: Prentice-Hall.

Gross, D. R., & Capuzzi, D. (1998). Group counseling stages and issues. D. Capuzzi & D. R. Gross (Eds.). *Introduction to group counseling* (2nd ed.) (pp. 31–46). Denver, CO: Love Publishing.

Johnson, D. W., & Johnson, F. P. (1997). Group Dynamics. *Joining together: Group theory and group skills* (6th ed.) (pp. 3–47). Boston: Allyn and Bacon.

Johnson, D. W., & Johnson, F. P. (1997). Stage development of learning groups. *Joining together: Group theory and group skills* (6th ed.) (pp. 469–474). Boston: Allyn and Bacon.

Morganett, R. S. (1990). Guidelines for group success. *Skills for life: Group counseling activities for young adolescents* (pp. 7–10). Champaign, IL: Research Press.

Napier, R. W., Gershenfeld, M. K. (1993). A preliminary theory of norm development. *Groups: Theory and experience* (5th ed.) (pp. 140–143). Boston: Houghton Mifflin.

Napier, R. W., Gershenfeld, M. K. (1993). How group norms develop. *Groups: Theory and experience* (5th ed.) (pp. 22–126). Boston: Houghton Mifflin.

Napier, R. W., Gershenfeld, M. K. (1993). The evolution of groups. *Groups: Theory and experience* (5th ed.) (pp. 475–519). Boston: Houghton Mifflin.

Peck, M. S., (1987). Patterns of transformation. *The different drum: Community making and peace* (pp. 186–208). New York: Simon and Schuster.

Schmuck, R. A., Schmuck, P. A. (1997). Group development. *Group processes in the classroom* (7th ed.) (pp. 2–31). Madison, WI: Brown & Benchmark.

Weiner, M. F. (1984). Starting a group. *Techniques of group psychotherapy* (pp. 151–159). Washington, DC: American Psychiatric Press.

Weiner, M. F. (1984). Termination. *Techniques of group psychotherapy* (pp. 215–230). Washington, DC: American Psychiatric Press.

Weiner, M. F. (1984). The group process. *Techniques of group psychotherapy* (pp. 55–76). Washington, DC: American Psychiatric Press.

Yalom, I. D. (1983). A consistent, coherent group procedure. *Inpatient group psychotherapy* (pp. 120–123). New York: Basic Books.

Yalom, I. D. (1995). The advanced group. *The theory and practice of group psychotherapy* (4th ed.) (pp. 326–368). New York: Basic Books.

Yalom, I. D. (1995). The therapist's task in the here-and-now. *The theory and practice of group psychotherapy* (4th ed.) (pp. 139–143). New York: Basic Books.

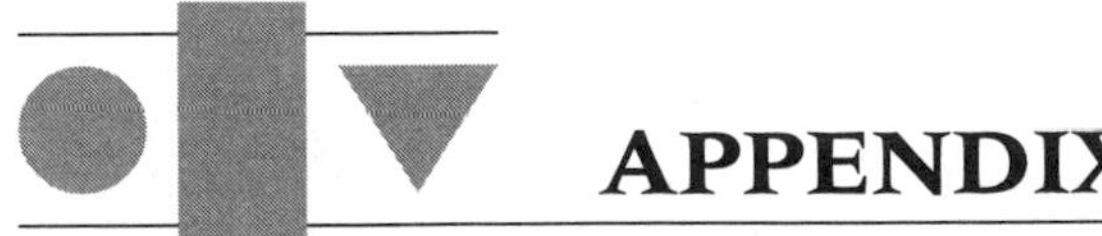

APPENDIX C

CD-ROM ReadMe Windows

Below you will find information about the CD-ROM, which includes the following:

Basics
Running this application
Video performance and system requirements
QuickTime installation
Printing and saving files
Accessing the Web site
Known bugs

Basics

You need a computer running Microsoft Windows95 or Windows98 operating systems. You should not run any other programs while you are running BCRG. The computer should be, at the minimum, a 120-mhz Pentium. Digital video is demanding. The faster the computer, the better the performance.

The computer needs

- A CD drive (minimum 8-speed, the faster the better)
- A Sound Blaster 16-bit-compatible sound card
- Speakers or headphones
- A color monitor capable of 16-bit color (thousands)
- At least 24 mb of RAM (more is better)
- A hard drive or floppy disk to save answers and print files

To get the best color, set your display or monitor to 16-bit (thousands) color. Look for Display in your Control Panels. (On the Windows desktop, select Start and then Settings.) If video performance is sluggish, you may want to set the color depth to 256 or 8-bit. The color will not be as good, but the video will run better.

Make sure the volume of your sound card is set to an audible range. (Look for the audio tab in Multimedia in your Control Panels.) There is volume control inside BCRG, but it is better to start with the system volume set in the upper 30 percent range.

Running This Application

In order to run this application, you must have Apple Computer's QuickTime 4 installed on your system. If you do, double-click on the program icon, BCRG.exe. This will start the program.

If you don't have QuickTime installed (or if you have an earlier version of it), you must install it. See the section "QuickTime Installation" below.

After you have installed QuickTime, start the application by double-clicking on BCRG.exe.

Video Performance and System Requirements

The digital video is compressed, using the Sorenson algorithm. This algorithm produces very high-quality video images but requires a 120- to 140-mhz Pentium II–class computer to work effectively. If your computer is below this CPU speed, you will experience "jerkiness" in the playback of the video. In Apple's QuickTime, the audio stream is given priority in playback, and if the computer begins to fall behind, video frames are dropped to keep up with the audio. We recommend that you have no other programs running while you are using this application (except for the Web browser). Playback can also be improved when observing sessions by selecting "hide" for the response, intent, and focus.

The operating system requirement is Windows 95 or Windows 98. Windows 2000 is not supported. Additional requirements are 16 mb of available RAM (above operating system usage), a Sound Blaster–compatible sound card with headphones or speakers, and a color display with thousands (16-bit) of colors.

QuickTime Installation

There are installers on this disk to install QuickTime. Find and open the folder Install QuickTime 4.1. You will see two choices for the installation.

If you are not connected to the Internet, you must use the installer located in the folder: QuickTime standalone installer. Open the folder and double-click on the installer, QuickTime, Installer.exe and follow the instructions.

If you are connected to the Internet, you have two choices for installation. You can use the standalone installer as above, or you can install QuickTime directly from Apple Computer's Web site. Open the folder Install QT from Apple Web site and double-click on QuickTimeInstaller.exe. The advantage in choosing the Web site installation method is that you may get a more up-to-date version of QuickTime. As of April 13, 2000, the most recent version is on this disk as the "standalone" installer.

Printing and Saving Files

You can print your exercise work and notes directly from BCRG if you have access to a printer from your computer. The option to print is presented first when you "save work" in an exercise. If you do not have a printer, you may want to save your work to a floppy disk for printing later on a PC with access to a printer.

The option to save to disk is presented second when you "save work" in an exercise. By default, three files are created and are named as follows:

1. BCRGx.TXT—a print file containing your exercise answers
2. BCRGxNotes.TXT—a print file containing your notes
3. BCRGx.BCR—an answer file for resuming the exercise using Get Work (where x is the exercise number)

The text files (1 and 2) are for your use. You can load them into a word-processing application such as Microsoft Word to edit and print them. Instructions for doing this follow. You may delete them at any time if you wish. The answer file (*.BCR) should never be edited; you can delete it when you know you will no longer want to resume work on the exercise in BCRG.

When you save work to disk in BCRG, a standard file-save dialog window will be presented. The first time you save after entering BCRG, the computer is "pointed at" the CD-ROM disk drive. Because you cannot save files to the CD-ROM disk (it is a read-only disk), you must point the computer at a different disk for saving. You do this using the buttons at the top of the dialog box; normally you will want to either save to the hard drive (often the drive called C:) or a floppy (often the drive called A:); the disk designations on your computer may be different. You may wish to save in a folder on your hard drive such as My Documents or you may wish to create a folder such as BCRG Work just for these documents. It is important to remember where you saved so that you can find your work to print it or to resume BCRG later.

As mentioned above, BCRG uses a default naming convention of BCRGx.*, where x is the exercise number. You can change the name if you wish (for example, you might want to add "partial" or "complete" to the end of the name). Do not add a file extension (the part to the right of the "dot") to your file name or include any dots in the file name itself. It is okay to save to the same file name repeatedly if you wish.

To print the text files (1 and 2 above), you can double-click on a file to open the default text editor on your machine. This default editor will have a rudimentary print option. Be sure to choose the Word Wrap option if available on the Edit menu to improve the appearance of the printed file.

For best results, print these text files from a word-processing application where you can edit and format them as you wish. To do this, first run the word-processing application (such as Word). Then choose the File Open command, and be sure the option is selected to open Files of type: All Files (*.*). This will allow you to see your BCRG files from the word-processing application. Go to the disk and folder where you stored your files (again using the buttons at the top of the dialog box). Once there, select the *.TXT file (either exercise work or notes) to open. Edit, format, and print the file; you can save the word-processing version of your file if you wish, although it is not necessary.

Accessing the Web Site

In order for the Web link to work, you must have Microsoft's Internet Explorer or Netscape's Navigator installed and have an Internet connection. The Basic Counseling Responses in Groups Web site is located at:

http://helpingprofs.wadsworth.com/haney_leibBCRG/index.html

BCRG will launch your Web browser when you click the Web button. If your Web browser is set up to connect to the Internet automatically when it is launched, you will be connected. If your Web browser is not set up to automatically connect, you will need to establish the connection to the Internet before running BCRG.

Known Bugs

On the exercise screen, you may have to click the play button on the video controller two or three times to replay the video under certain circumstances.

Portions of the video window-display rectangle flash when certain BCRG buttons are clicked or actions are taken. Though irritating, this has no adverse impact on the operation of BCRG or video playback.

In the exercises, every effort was made to stop the session videos at the end of complete sentences spoken by the counselors and clients. In a few unavoidable cases, a word or two may have been lost or added when the video stopped.

On the Macintosh, an intermittent problem has been seen while playing the video. During Observe or while doing the exercises, the video may stop and an alert may or may not appear that says "Property not found: #movieTime." The audio often continues, but the computer is unable to control BCRG (it may appear locked or frozen). To exit, enter Command-Q on the Mac. This problem has not been seen on the PC, but should it occur, enter Ctrl-Q to exit. Reboot the computer, and reenter BCRG. If you experience this problem on your system, save your exercise work often.

On some older Macs, the Introduction cannot be interrupted. There is currently no workaround for this problem. The Introduction lasts approximately three minutes.

CD-ROM ReadMe Macintosh

You may be able to listen to this information. Look at the menu at the top of the screen. If you see Sound, see if there is a Speak All option. If there is, you can select it and choose your voice. If not, you'll just have to read it.

Below you will find information about this CD-ROM, which includes the following:

Basics
Running this application
Video performance and system requirements
QuickTime installation
Printing and saving files
Accessing the Web site
Known bugs

Basics

You need an Apple Macintosh PowerPC running system 7.5.3 or later. You should not run any other programs while you are running BCRG. The computer should be, at the minimum, a 120-mhz PowerPC. Digital video is demanding. The faster the computer, the better the performance.

The computer needs

- A CD drive and should be at least a 8x-speed drive
- Speakers or a headset
- A color monitor capable of 16-bit (thousands) color
- At least 12 mb of available RAM (more is better)—the part that the system is not using

To get the best color, set your display or monitor to 16-bit (thousands) color. Look in Monitors & Sound in your Control Panels under the Apple icon in the upper left corner of your screen. If video performance is sluggish, you may want to set the color depth to 256 or 8-bit. The color will not be as good, but the video will run better.

Make sure your system volume is set to an audible range. Look in Monitors & Sound in your Control Panels under the Apple icon in the upper left corner of your screen. There is volume control inside BCRG, but it is better to start with the system volume set in the upper 30 percent range.

Running This Application

In order to run this application, you must have Apple Computer's QuickTime 4 installed on your system. If you do, double-click on the program icon, BCRG. This will start the program.

If you don't have QuickTime installed (or if you have an earlier version of it), you must install it. See the section "QuickTime Installation" below.

After you have installed QuickTime, start the application by double-clicking on BCRG.

Video Performance and System Requirements

The digital video is compressed, using the Sorenson algorithm. This algorithm produces very high-quality video images, but requires a 120- to 140-mhz PowerMac computer to work effectively. If your computer runs below this cpu speed, you will experience "jerkiness" in the playback of the video. In Apple's QuickTime, the audio stream is given priority in playback, and if the computer begins to fall behind, video frames are dropped to keep up with the audio. We recommend that you have no other programs running while you are using this application (except for the Web browser). Playback can also be improved when observing sessions by selecting "hide" for the response, intent, and focus.

Additional requirements are Mac O/S 7.5.3 or later and 12mb of available system memory (in addition to what is used by the operating system).

QuickTime Installation

There are installers on this disk to install QuickTime. Find and open the folder Install QuickTime 4.1. You will see two choices for the installation.

If you are not connected to the Internet, you must use the installer located in the folder: QuickTime standalone installer. Open the folder and double-click on the installer, QuickTime Installer, and follow the instructions.

If you are connected to the Internet, you have two choices for installation. You can use the standalone installer as above, or you can install QuickTime directly from Apple Computer's Web site. Open the folder Install QT from Apple Web site and double-click on QuickTime Installer. The advantage in choosing the Web-site installation method is that you may get a more up-to-date version of QuickTime. As of April 13, 2000, the most recent version is on this disk as the "standalone" installer.

Printing and Saving Files

You can print your exercise work and notes directly from BCRG if you have access to a printer from your computer. The option to print is presented first when you "save work" in an exercise. If you do not have a printer, you may want to save your work to a floppy disk for printing later on a Mac with access to a printer.

The option to save to disk is presented second when you "save work" in an exercise. By default, three files are created and are named as follows:

1. BCRGx.TXT—a print file containing your exercise answers
2. BCRGxNotes.TXT—a print file containing your notes
3. BCRGx.BCR—an answer file for resuming the exercise, using Get Work (where x is the exercise number)

The text files (1 and 2) are for your use. You can load them into a word-processing application such as Microsoft Word to edit and print them. Instructions for doing this follow. You may delete them at any time if you wish. The answer file (*.BCR) should never be edited; you can delete it when you know you will no longer want to resume work on the exercise in BCRG.

When you save work in BCRG, a standard file-save dialog window will be presented. The first time you save after entering BCRG, the computer is "pointed at" the CD-ROM drive. As you cannot save files to the CD-ROM (it is a read-only disk), you must point the computer at a different disk for saving. You do this using the buttons at the top of the dialog box; normally you will want to either save to the hard drive or a floppy. It is important to remember where you saved so that you can find your work to print it or to resume BCRG later.

As mentioned above, BCRG uses a default naming convention of BCRGx.*, where x is the exercise number. You can change the name if you wish (for example, you might want to add "partial" or "complete" to the end of the name). Do not add a file extension (the part to the right of the "dot") to your file name or include any dots in the file name itself. It is okay to save to the same file name repeatedly.

To print the text files (1 and 2 above), you can double-click on a file to open the default text editor on your machine. This default editor will have a rudimentary print option. Be sure to choose the Word Wrap option if available on the Edit menu to improve the appearance of the printed file.

For best results, print these text files from a word-processing application where you can edit and format them as you wish. To do this, first run the word-processing application (such as Word). Then choose the File Open command, and be sure the option is selected to open Files of type: All Files (*.*). This will allow you to see your BCRG files from the word-processing application. Go to the disk and folder where you stored your files (again using the buttons at the top of the dialog box). Once there, select the *.TXT file (either exercise work or notes) to open. Edit, format, and print the file; you can save the word-processing version of your file if you wish, although it is not necessary.

Accessing the Web Site

In order for the Web link to work, you must have Microsoft's Internet Explorer or Netscape's Navigator installed and have an Internet connection. The Basic Counseling Responses in Groups Web site is located at:

http://helpingprofs.wadsworth.com/haney_leibBCRG/index.html

BCRG will launch your Web browser when you click the Web button. If your Web browser is set up to connect to the Internet automatically when it is launched, you will be connected. If your Web browser is not set up to automatically connect, you will need to establish the connection to the Internet before running BCRG.

Known Bugs

On the exercise screen, you may have to click the play button on the video controller two or three times to replay the video under certain circumstances.

Portions of the video window-display rectangle flash when certain BCRG buttons are clicked or actions are taken. Though irritating, this has no adverse impact on the operation of BCRG or video playback.

In the exercises, every effort was made to stop the session videos at the end of complete sentences spoken by the counselors and clients. In a few unavoidable cases, a word or two may have been lost or added when the video stopped.

On the Macintosh, an intermittent problem has been seen while playing the video. During Observe or while doing the exercises, the video may stop and an alert may or may not appear that says "Property not found: #movieTime." The audio often continues, but the computer is unable to control BCRG (it may appear locked or frozen). To exit, enter Command-Q on the Mac. This problem has not been seen on the PC, but should it occur, enter Ctrl-Q to exit. Reboot the computer, and reenter BCRG. If you experience this problem on your system, save your exercise work often.

On some older Macs, the introduction cannot be interrupted. There is currently no workaround for this problem. The introduction lasts approximately three minutes.

CD-ROM Help

Basic Counseling Responses in Groups

Since the Select Screen is where you start, this is a logical place to explain how the CD-ROM functions in general. The buttons on the bottom of the screen are for "getting around." When you roll your cursor over them, a cue is given about their function. For example, E is Do Exercise; once you have selected a group on the Select screen, click E to do the exercise featuring that group. Likewise, click O to observe the group.

On each of the screens, you will notice that different buttons are shown on the right side of the screen. The select screen has seven buttons in all: the buttons numbered 1 through 5 allow you to select a group; the Replay Intro button allows you to watch the Intro again; and the Describe button plays an audio description of the selected group. The selected group is clearly identified.

You can return to the select screen at any time if you want to switch from one group to another; simply click on the new group number you want to observe or to focus on for the exercise.

Observing Groups

The Observe Screen allows you to observe the selected group video from start to finish. The group video will begin playing automatically when you enter this screen. Use the video control bar under the video display area to control playback much as you would the buttons on a VCR. Click on the horizontal scroll bar to quickly position the group video at any point of interest.

By default, when the counselor speaks, the response, intent, and focus of the counselor response will be shown under the video window. If you do not wish to see the response, intent, and focus while you are playing the video, click the Hide button on the right side of the observe screen. To show it again, simply click Show.

When showing the response, intent, and focus, you may notice that the video playback is not as smooth. This is normal. If you find it unpleasant, click Hide.

Viewing Examples

The View Examples Screen allows you to view examples of the fifteen responses, three intents, and group-related focuses. Examples are taken from the group videos. Only the counselor response is shown.

To view an example, click on one of the three buttons on the right side of the screen: View Response, View Intent, or View Focus. A list to choose from is then displayed to the right of the video screen. To view an example, click on the item in the list. The response, intent, and focus of the counselor response are displayed under the video window as the example is played.

Exercise 1

Use the Exercise screen to complete the exercise featuring Group 1/Women. The CD-ROM guides you through the exercise by stopping the video for you at appropriate times and by presenting buttons on the right side when needed. Click Proceed to start the exercise.

Exercise 1 stops *after* eight selected counselor responses. The verbatim counselor response and the RESPONSE, intent, and focus are shown. You should:

1. Click Create to create a response with a *different focus* than the one chosen by the counselor. Simply begin typing; your response will appear in the student-counselor response area.
2. Click Compare to compare your response to other possibilities.
3. Click Proceed to move on to the next series of interactions.

To print your exercise work and notes at any time, click Save Work and answer Yes when asked if you want to print your work now (if you cannot access a printer from your computer, click No). You are then asked if you want to save your work and notes to a disk file. Save your work only if you want to finish it, review it, or print it later (Get Work). For more information about saving files to disk, see the Readme file on the CD-ROM.

Exercise 2

Use the Exercise screen to complete the exercise featuring Group 2/Boys. The CD-ROM guides you through the exercise by stopping the video for you at appropriate times and by presenting buttons on the right side when needed. Click Proceed to start the exercise.

Exercise 2 stops *after* thirteen selected counselor responses. The verbatim counselor response and the RESPONSE, intent, and focus are shown. You should:

1. Click Create to create a response with a *different focus* than the one chosen by the counselor. Simply begin typing; your response will appear in the student-counselor response area.

2. Click Compare to compare your response to other possibilities.
3. Click Proceed to move on to the next series of interactions.

To print your exercise work and notes at any time, click Save Work and answer Yes when asked if you want to print your work now (if you cannot access a printer from your computer, click No). You are then asked if you want to save your work and notes to a disk file. Save your work only if you want to finish it, review it, or print it later (Get Work). For more information about saving files to disk, see the Readme file on the CD-ROM.

Exercise 3

Use the Exercise screen to complete the exercise featuring Group 3/Graduates. The CD-ROM guides you through the exercise by stopping the video for you at appropriate times, and by presenting buttons on the right side when needed. Click Proceed to start the exercise.

Exercise 3 stops just *before* eight selected counselor responses. You should:

1. Click Identify Response to select the response you wish to use at this point. Likewise, click Identify Intent to select the intent. Click Identify Focus to select the focus; note that a complete focus must include a "who" and a "what" and may include a "where" and/or "when."
2. Click Create to create a response that demonstrates the response, intent, and focus you just selected.
3. Click Compare to compare your response to the verbatim counselor response and the corresponding RESPONSE, intent, and focus.
4. Click Proceed to move on to the next series of interactions.

To print your exercise work and notes at any time, click Save Work and answer Yes when asked if you want to print your work now (if you cannot access a printer from your computer, click No). You are then asked if you want to save your work and notes to a disk file. Save your work only if you want to finish it, review it, or print it later (Get Work). For more information about saving files to disk, see the Readme file on the CD-ROM.

Exercise 4

Use the Exercise screen to complete the exercise featuring Group 4/Students. The CD-ROM guides you through the exercise by stopping the video for you at appropriate times and by presenting buttons on the right side when needed. Click Proceed to start the exercise.

Exercise 4 stops just *before* ten selected counselor responses. You should:

1. Click Identify Response to select the response you wish to use at this point. Likewise, click Identify Intent to select the intent. Click Identify Focus to select the focus; note that a complete focus must include a "who" and a "what" and may include a "where" and/or "when."
2. Click Create to create a response that demonstrates the response, intent, and focus you just selected.
3. Click Compare to compare your response to the verbatim counselor response and the corresponding RESPONSE, intent, and focus.
4. Click Proceed to move on to the next series of interactions.

To print your exercise work and notes at any time, click Save Work and answer Yes when asked if you want to print your work now (if you cannot access a printer from your computer, click No). You are then asked if you want to save your work and notes to a disk file. Save your work only if you want to finish it, review it, or print it later (Get Work). For more information about saving files to disk, see the Readme file on the CD-ROM.

Exercise 5

Use the Exercise screen to complete the exercise featuring Group 5/Adults. The CD-ROM guides you through the exercise by stopping the video for you at appropriate times and by presenting buttons on the right side when needed. Click Proceed to start the exercise.

Exercise 5 stops just *before* eleven selected counselor responses. You should:

1. Click Create to create a response that you wish to make at this point.
2. Identify the response you just made. Click Identify Response to select the response. Likewise, click Identify Intent to select the intent. Click Identify Focus to select the focus; note that a complete focus must include a "who" and a "what" and may include a "where" and/or "when."
3. Click Compare to compare your response to the verbatim counselor response and the corresponding RESPONSE, intent, and focus.
4. Click Proceed to move on to the next series of interactions.

To print your exercise work and notes at any time, click Save Work and answer Yes when asked if you want to print your work now (if you cannot access a printer from your computer, click No). You are then asked if you want to save your work and notes to a disk file. Save your work only if you want to finish it, review it, or print it later (Get Work). For more information about saving files to disk, see the Readme file on the CD-ROM.

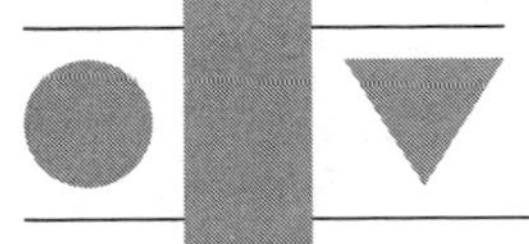

REFERENCES

Carroll, M. R., & Wiggins, J. D. (1997). *Elements of group counseling: Back to the basics* (2nd ed.). Denver, CO: Love Publishing.

Corey, G. (2000). *Theory and practice of group counseling* (5th ed.). Pacific Grove, CA: Brooks/Cole-Wadsworth.

Gladding, S. T. (1999). *Group work: A counseling specialty* (3rd ed.). Upper Saddle River, NJ: Prentice-Hall.

Haney, H., & Leibsohn, J. (1999). *Basic counseling responses.* Pacific Grove, CA: Brooks/Cole-Wadsworth.

Ivey, Allen E., Pedersen, Paul B., Ivey, Mary Bradford (2001). *Intentional group counseling, a microskills approach.* Pacific Grove, CA: Brooks/Cole-Wadsworth.

Jacobs, E. E., Masson, R. L. & Harvill, R. L. (1998). *Group counseling: Strategies and skills* (3rd ed.). Pacific Grove, CA: Brooks/Cole-Wadsworth.

Kottler, J. A. (1994). *Advanced group leadership.* Pacific Grove, CA: Brooks/Cole-Wadsworth.

Morganett, R. S. (1990). *Skills for life: Group counseling activities for young adolescents.* Champaign, IL: Research Press.

Peck, F. Scott. (1987). *A different drum.* New York: Simon and Schuster.

Reid, Kenneth E. (1997). *Social work practice with groups: A clinical perspective.* Pacific Grove, CA: Brooks/Cole-Wadsworth.

Yalom, I. D. (1995). *The theory and practice of group psychotherapy* (4th ed.). New York: Basic Books.

Zastrow, Charles (1996). *Social work with groups* (4th ed.). Chicago: Nelson-Hall, Inc.

INDEX

TO THE OWNER OF THIS PACKAGE

We are very interested in learning more about how you are using the components of *Basic Counseling Responses™ in Groups* (worktext, videocassette, and CD-ROM with Web links). Please take a moment to fill out this MULTI-MEDIA SURVEY:

Name:____________________ **School:** ____________________
Course: ____________________ **E-mail:** ____________________
Instructor: ____________________

1. Are you using all the components of this package? If not, which are you using and why? Which have you not used yet, and why?
2. Please share your impressions of this package? How is it helping you to learn? How could it be even better?
3. Do you have easy access to a VCR? ❍ Yes ❍ No
   If yes, is it your own VCR or the property of the school
4. Do you have easy access to a computer? ❍ Yes ❍ No
   If yes, is it your own computer or the property of the school?
5. Do you have access to computer labs for learning concepts in specific coursework? ❍ Yes ❍ No
   If yes, which courses? ____________________
   Instructor(s): ____________________
6. How many computer labs are available? ❍ 0 ❍ 1 ❍ 2 ❍ 3 ❍ 4 ❍ 5 ❍ Greater than 5 How many? _____
7. How many computers, on average, are in each of these labs?
   ❍ <10 ❍ 10–20 ❍ 21–30 ❍ 31–50 ❍ 51–100 ❍ > 100
8. Are any of these labs for the exclusive use of your program's department? ❍ Yes ❍ No
   If yes, how many computers do you have exclusive department rights to? _____
   If no, what other departments do you share with?
   ❍ Sociology ❍ Psychology ❍ Education ❍ Other: ____________________
9. How are you currently using your computer lab(s)? (check as many as apply)
   ❍ For free time, to complete assignments/homework
   ❍ Used during designated computer lab time, access to technology products/tools to complete specific assignments
   ❍ Primary location where your classes meet
   ❍ You don't use the computer lab(s)
   ❍ Other: ____________________
10. What operating system do you use personally?
    ❍ Win 95 ❍ Win 3.1 ❍ Win NT ❍ Macintosh ❍ Unix ❍ OS2 ❍ Mix of Win and Mac
11. What is the current dominant operating system in your computer lab(s)?
    ❍ Win 95 ❍ Win 3.1 ❍ Win NT ❍ Macintosh ❍ Unix ❍ OS2 ❍ Mix of Win and Mac
12. What operating system do think will be dominant in two years?
    ❍ Win 98 ❍ Win 95 ❍ Win 3.1 ❍ Win NT ❍ Macintosh ❍ Unix ❍ OS2
13. When do you think technology will be used by a majority of your instructors as part of their course(s)?
    ❍ Never ❍ 1998 ❍ 1999 ❍ 2000 ❍ 2001 ❍ 2002 ❍ > 2002 ❍ A majority already is
14. Do you currently use the Web in your course(s)? ❍ Yes ❍ No If yes, how are you using the Web?
    ❍ To obtain raw data for various assignments and labs
    ❍ To find information on topics discussed in class or discovered in this package
    ❍ To access information from a textbook publisher's Web server
    ❍ To access information from a software publisher's Web server
    ❍ For a distance/distributed learning environment where some students are off-site/not in your classroom
    ❍ Other: ____________________

Any other comments?

OPTIONAL:

Your name: ______________________________ Date: ________________

May Wadsworth quote you, either in promotion for *Basic Counseling Responses™ in Groups*, or in future publishing ventures?

Yes: _________ No: _________

Sincerely yours,

Hutch Haney

Jacqueline Leibsohn

FOLD HERE

NO P
NEC
IF M
IN
UNITE

BUSINESS REPLY MAIL

FIRST CLASS PERMIT NO. 358 PACIFIC GROVE, CA

POSTAGE WILL BE PAID BY ADDRESSEE

ATTN: Counseling Editor, Lisa Gebo

WADSWORTH/THOMSON LEARNING
511 FOREST LODGE ROAD
PACIFIC GROVE, CA 93950-9968

FOLD HERE